Praise for the book, *Despite L*

Lupus is a life-altering disease. What Sara [Gorman] learned is that she could let lupus alter her life or she could take charge and alter her own life to achieve better control of her lupus. During the struggle that she shares with her readers, she acquired the wisdom to accept that she would live the rest of her life with lupus. She also developed the courage to rebuild her life with lupus by taking charge of what she could control, and she shares that story. Those elements of wisdom, acceptance and taking control underlie many if not most of the stories that I hear of successfully living with lupus, and that is why I hope many will read Sara's story and learn from its message of hope.

–Penny Fletcher, President and CEO
Lupus Foundation of America
Greater Washington Chapter

Sara [Gorman] has written a gem of a book for lupus patients struggling with a new, frightening and unpredictable illness. Her advice is also applicable to all of us: lead a healthier, happier life. Discover the inner self and what is really important to you. Change is the cornerstone of life. Sometimes when we are feeling awful, we fear that "I will feel like this forever". That feeling is understandable but completely false. Things always change. Knowing that we will not feel the same the next day or the next week is comforting. Our ability to change and put our happiness and the happiness of our loved ones as the core of our existence makes us happier and healthier people with our chronic disease, whatever that disease may be. Sara's book helps us learn these and other truths to help us live with lupus and lead happier lives.

–Neil I. Stahl, MD
Rheumatologist

An invaluable resource for those dealing, not just with lupus, but any chronic illness. Truly moving.

–Sam Rogers
Alliance for Lupus Research

Suffering through a chronic illness can be one of life's great challenges. Not only do you have to deal with the physical ailment, but you also have to work through the emotional struggle that goes along with it. Then there's the "what if's": "What if we never find a cure?" "What if I never get better?" "What if I'm sick the rest of my life?" And there's also the pressure it can put on relationships. Sara Gorman experienced all of these — and was able to come through victoriously. Her story is inspiring, challenging, and, most importantly, full of hope for anyone diagnosed with Lupus or any chronic illness.

–Steve Kroening
Freelance writer for Success magazine
Publisher of wisdomsedge.com

Praise for the blog, DESPITELUPUS.COM

"...as a fellow lupie, I have to tell you how remarkable it is to finally have found someone who can communicate the frustrations and challenges of this diagnosis." - Anonymous

"I have RA, but a lot of the things you write about are universal to chronic diseases, so I get a lot out of your posts." — S.

"I've never known anyone with lupus so I have felt very alone and frustrated. I am enjoying your honesty. It's nice to read about someone who is dealing with it instead of it dealing with them." — K.

"...reading your blog has definitely kept me doing the right things...Thanks for your positive outlook, it helps me keep my chin up..." - M.P.

"...You are right on so many points in this post. Funny, how much of what you went through and still are that I relate to, even though yours is a chronic illness and mine was acute." — Deborah Ludwig, author of Rebirth: A Leukemia Survivor's Journal of Healing during Chemotherapy, Bone Marrow Transplant, and Recovery

"...You express what I feel so well...It's so nice to know [this] isn't something I'm experiencing alone." - A.

"I will have to keep an eye out for your book. I enjoy reading your blog as I can really relate to [many] of the feelings you have about things...Kudos to you girlfriend! " - M. N. V.

"...I am finding it to be a good practice to look at your blog...for a sanity check and just to remind myself to slow down and be more careful about what I get involved with...It's great (even for a non-lupite)!" — J.H.

"I just love reading your stuff - and am amazed at your strength and humor. Thank you for being out there for all of us." - M.P.

"... I can't wait to read the book! You provide wonderful insights and great resources for people." — G.V.

"Your blog is fantastic! You are an excellent writer -- I found myself really drawn in, and wanting to read more. Even though I don't have Lupus, I felt I could really relate to much of what you write about." — R.C.

"Wow, I just read your whole blog and I feel like we are leading almost identical lives." - M.

"I've been following your journey for several months and I find you to be inspirational." — D.C.

"...What a wonderful woman, fighter and awesome writer..." — S.

"Thanks for sharing the recommendations! It's always good to find new ways of helping to deal with the pain." — C.

"I read your blog and I find that you are such a strong person...thanks for sharing." — A.Z.

"Your poem is awesome and says EXACTLY how I feel. You nailed it girl! Good job!" - M.P.

"Great blog, your profile inspired me. I have lupus & I too have been fighting life." — M.M.

"Sometimes your blog serves as a reminder that I'm doing too much! ...I definitely need to be better at recognizing the fatigue before I get really sick!" — L.B.

"Your insights show a [lot] of personal growth and reflection - someone who lives with the disease and seeks to understand its role in our life and relationships." — C.J.

"Excellent blog...you are a hero!" — A.C.

"I enjoyed reading your blog - thanks for sharing! Your story is inspiring." — S.T.

"It's informative, well written, and colorful...your stories are powerful." — M.S.

"Your blog is great. The entries have a great balance of information and the casualness of talking to a friend." — S.F.

"...Just wanted you to know how interesting it is to read your stories and how amazing your attitude and personality [are] in spite of all that you've been through and continue to go through." — C.T.

"You are such an exceptional writer, and your stories are so moving..." - E.H.

"I really respect your blog...It's good to hear from someone out there that has lupus [and] is pregnant and having a positive experience... I think it is really helpful to know that there are other people out there just like me...you never get to hear about the good cases of lupus and pregnancy...you always only hear about the bad ones..." - A.W.

"I very much appreciate the blog - your writing, sharing, and providing it as a resource. There aren't enough good sites out there. Believe me, I've looked!" — M.T.

"...your blog is so great. I really enjoyed your writing. Everything is so well written; and very inspirational as well." — L.

"First of all, I want to thank you for the positive and comprehensive review you wrote in the first blog! It was one of the best I've ever seen! And then the second one, in which you expressed some valid concerns, was also very well done, factual and comprehensive. I truly appreciate that..." — R.C.

"Thanks for this post. It's good to hear reminders like this from time to time." — S.

despite

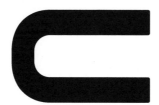
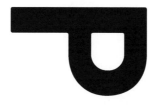
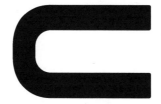
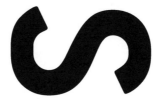

DESPITE LUPUS

How to Live Well with a Chronic Illness

PUBLISHER
Four-Legged Press

ISBN
978-1-4392-3489-1

Library of Congress Control Number
2009903955

BOOK COVER
Cecilia Sorochin · SoroDesign
cover photograph by Vladimir Kozeev
author photograph by Erica Vinyard

BOOK DESIGN
Cecilia Sorochin · SoroDesign

TYPESET
Filosofia by Zuzana Licko
ITC Conduit by Mark van Bronkhorst

www.despitelupus.com

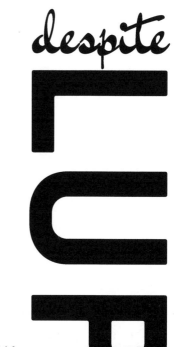

despite

LUPUS

HOW
TO
LIVE
WELL
WITH
A
CHRONIC
ILLNESS

SARA GORMAN

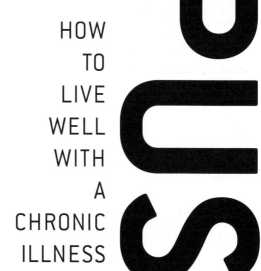

Acknowledgements

I've been surrounded by encouraging people since the day I was diagnosed with lupus, and that support has continued throughout the process of writing this book. Here are just a few of the people who have helped me reach my goals of living well with lupus and then choosing to write about it:

To my editor, Sara Ford Burstein, who was an invaluable resource throughout the entire editing process. From the table of contents to the endnotes and everything in between, Sara significantly improved the manuscript without changing its message. I was thrilled that she was the first one to read the text and honored to have worked with such a perceptive, insightful, talented person!

To Dr. Neil Stahl, who has worked so hard to make me better and who continues to keep me well. I hope every lupus patient can find a remarkable rheumatologist like the one I did. To Dr. George Bazaco, my pulmonologist, who was the first doctor to suggest that I be tested for lupus. He eased me into the concept of having a chronic illness, and continues to treat me as if I'm his only patient. To the doctors at Perinatal Associates of Northern Virginia, who took such good care of me before, during and even after my pregnancy. Baby Deirdre thanks you, too.

To the members of my support group, from whom I've learned so much. In particular, to Karen, Carla, Anne, Angela and Beth: thank you for sharing your experiences with me and making me believe I'd get better. To Gail McCurry, who graciously agreed to write my forward and always encourages me to share my story.

To my friends and co-workers at Henninger Media Services, who made it so easy for me to do the right thing, and to Eric, in particular, for letting me know it was okay to quit. What a wonderful place to have spent 10 years!

To Beth Rubin and Mark Stricherz, for their advice on writing and publishing a book. Thank you for sharing your expertise! To the talented Cecilia Sorochin and Jeff Barry, both of whom embraced my project and designed one heck of a book.

To Penny Fletcher & the Lupus Foundation office, for making me feel like my story was worth sharing to the lupus community at large. To Sam Rogers at Alliance for Lupus Research, Steve Kroening at Wisdom's Edge, and Dr. Daniel Wallace, for taking the time to read and comment on my book.

To Father John McBrearty, for reminding me of the vital role patience plays in the game of life. To Maureen and Jodie, for coming to my rescue on more than one occasion.

To my parents, for teaching me life's most valuable lessons, especially the one about loving myself enough to stay well. To my in-laws, Maureen and John, who treat me as if I'm one of their own (even if I'm not an original!)

To Katie, for being the greatest big sister anyone could ever ask for, even when little sister wasn't behaving very well. To my brother-in-law, Kevin – the one night in the emergency room is enough to earn you a mention, but everything else you have done over the years is pretty great, too.

To Johnny, for living the words, "in sickness and in health." You inspired me to do things I never thought I could, and helped me every step of the way. Thank you for your last-minute improvements to the book, for answering all of my questions over the past 8 ½ years, and for reminding me not to let writing a book about staying healthy get in the way of staying healthy. You are my all-time favorite, and I love you.

To Deirdre, for waiting to come into this world until the time was right. You were worth the wait.

To Johnny, for teaching me how to nap

To Katie, for forcing me to take a nap

To Henry, for never missing a nap

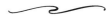

The unexpected journey...

TO BECOME WHO WE ARE, NOT JUST WHO WE WANT TO BE OR WHO WE WERE....

Once you meet Sara Gorman through her writing, you won't think about lupus or any other chronic illness in the same way. As a lupus support group facilitator, I witnessed some of her journey as a young woman, from newly married and newly diagnosed with lupus, to who she is today: a confident, new mother who has learned much about life and her illness.

There are few illnesses as frightening as lupus. Books and web sites have terrifying details about symptoms, quickly overwhelming anyone who reads them without the benefit of other supportive conversations. In fact, the process of understanding and healing comes best accompanied by open, flowing communication with medical care providers who specialize in treating lupus, others with lupus, family and close personal confidants. Common stories shared in support groups instruct and inspire while in-creased awareness, from any source, clarifies and stabilizes.

Inflammation and pain require immediate attention, but even when physical symp-toms are under control, fear can continue to drive decisions or impede progress. Even as Sara faced the worst, she knew it was possible to refocus her energies. We can see the result through her personal accounts contained in this book. Acceptance allowed her to look to the future and make other, better choices.

While individuals with lupus experience symptoms, they frequently look no different than they always have. This leads to difficulty understanding how they can feel so bad when they look so good. Family members, employers, co-workers and the public fre-quently misinterpret lupus symptoms because of this, yet lupus is a unique illness that can give those with lupus an altered sense of themselves and the world around them.

This is the unexpected journey for anyone with lupus. From first diagnoses through flares and remission, learning about lupus and accepting life as it is, is required. While physically and emotionally difficult and demanding at times, the effort to incorporate lupus into daily life brings its own important rewards. Sara provides a testament to her healing and to the support she received.

Listening to inner thoughts and feelings is not easy at any time of life, and it becomes much more complicated when dealing with lupus. Sara shows us that there are ways to develop an honest conversation with oneself and to transform difficult emotions, especially with the engaged support of others. The journey begins with honesty with oneself and continues with the process of reaching out to others to extend and soften that internal process. Healing comes both from within and without.

Sara's illness was diagnosed within a month of her symptoms, but many people with lupus have serious episodes of illness for some time before they are finally diagnosed. Some are diagnosed after having joint pain, fatigue and hair loss. Others have a rash and fatigue. Lupus presents itself in different ways, and individuals respond individually. Organs can be involved with lupus and people can experience what is commonly called "brain fog" or times when they feel foggy and unable to process as fluently as previously.

In this book, Sara offers a hard-fought sense about how she found her growing capacity and increased awareness. To Sara, what appeared to be weakness and defeat early in her disease became, later, strength from the acceptance and knowledge that she could better anticipate and manage, not only her life, but also her reaction to lupus. From spreadsheets to informed consultations with her doctor, Sara gradually gained knowledge and confidence, which she now shares with the reader.

For the first time, the reader who does not have lupus can understand the unpredictability of the illness and the debility of the symptoms. Those who have lupus can identify with Sara's pain and grief. And all can learn from her study of her own illness and her integration of important steps to healing.

What follows is Sara's unexpected journey, her hope, faith and courage along with her lessons in living.

With deepest respect,
Gail McCurry, LCSW
Alexandria Lupus Support Group Facilitator

15

Introduction

A year before I was diagnosed with Systemic Lupus Erythematosus ("SLE" or "lupus"), I met Susan[1], a young woman who had been suffering with the disease for several months. I was clueless about lupus at the time, and the description of her disease was shocking. From the onset of Susan's illness, she suffered terrible, arthritic pain throughout her entire body. Her joints were prone to massive swelling for days on end. She couldn't be exposed to the sun because it worsened her condition. She lost almost all of her hair. She had the remains of a severe rash across her nose and cheeks that was red and unsightly. She'd recently quit her job, postponed her wedding, and moved into her parent's home due to the great bouts of fatigue that left her unable to care for herself.

Just months earlier, she had been a spunky, energetic college graduate, ready to tackle the world. Now, she could barely walk a few feet without struggling. As I learned of her terrible situation, I thought of how miserable she must be. I couldn't imagine what it would feel like to be so helpless and broken. I remember thinking to myself that I would rather die than have an awful thing like that happen to me at such a young age.

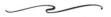

Less than a year later, at the age of 26, I suffered my first symptoms of lupus: chest pain, aching joints, sore throat, and a fever. The symptoms grew worse and more intense over the course of about three weeks, and within a month of experiencing those first symptoms, I was diagnosed with lupus. The lining around my lungs was filled with fluid, I was bed-ridden, and I shook constantly from the horrific pain. I was miserable, but the doctors told me I was lucky; at least we had identified the culprit.

I suffered terribly those first few months, taking one hit after another, never finding refuge from this new and ruthless enemy. I took a month off of work, had the fluid removed from my lungs twice, took more medication on a weekly basis than I had cumulatively taken in my whole life, and struggled to make it down six steps to the kitchen each morning. To say that life had changed was an understatement. I felt vulnerable and damaged, just as I envisioned Susan had a year before. But as sick as I was, I assumed lupus wouldn't affect me as deeply as it had touched her. I was stronger than she was, more determined, perhaps even better equipped to fight. A mere disease couldn't slow me down; I simply wouldn't let it.

THE FIGHT OF MY LIFE

At the time I was diagnosed, I had been married less than six weeks, was at a high point in my career in television production, and had no interest in letting a chronic illness upset my plans for the future. Therefore, I refused to let it do so. Yes, I was stuck with a confusing, chronic illness that was capable of inflicting debilitating pain and making me suffer miserably, but I decided to fight my way to wellness. I down-right revolted. I refused to give in to the disease, kicking and screaming every time lupus tried to assert herself. I thought my best defense was to deny the fact that I even had it, living with complete disregard to its limitations.

When I felt rundown or exhausted, I pushed on. When my joints were achy and swollen, I convinced myself they weren't and kept on moving. There were days when I was stuck in bed, severely sick and immobile, but most days, I just weathered the symptoms the best I could. I thought a positive attitude and an indomitable spirit would be the keys to coping with the physical and mental pain. If I didn't show any signs of weakness, lupus would take the hint and move on to someone more susceptible and defenseless. Those characteristics didn't fit my profile, and I was going do everything in my power to prevent lupus from changing me.

Unfortunately, lupus didn't care how hard I tried to fend off her symptoms. The more I pushed her away, the more she raged on. My symptoms worsened, and my health declined severely. I continued to believe that my determined efforts could be productive, if I just pushed a little harder. But my body didn't have anything more to give. The count-less medicines and pain killers, a blood transfusion, lung taps, multiple visits to the emergency room and a week in the hospital weren't enough to keep my body afloat anymore. Unlike any other adversary I'd ever been up against, lupus is a potentially fatal, chronic illness, and I was losing the battle.

For four years, I desperately struggled to keep hold of the life I'd known (demanding, yet fulfilling career, busy social life, packed vacation schedule, invincible attitude), but my body couldn't take it anymore. I was fighting life, instead of living it, and had resigned myself to the fact that I would be lucky if my body held out to the age of thirty.

I told myself I wasn't giving up; my body was just giving out, and there wasn't anything I could do about it. I began thinking about the things I should do before I died: work less; live more; appreciate my family; enjoy time with friends; be more creative; attempt to fulfill my personal, life-long goals in the limited time I had. The all-encompassing objective was to realign my priorities and get the most out of life, while I still could.

But as I crafted my plan for a premature death, it seemed I was making an even more compelling case for life. Why shouldn't I get my priorities in line right now, not for death's sake, but for the benefit of my future? Did I really have to work as much as I did, or was I letting pride and stubbornness rule my decision to do so? As committed as I was to acting as if lupus had left me unaffected, who was I keeping up appearances for, and was I profiting from the charade? I wanted to travel the world, have children, and enjoy my hobbies, but if I didn't start taking care of myself, I'd see none of those things come to pass.

It took me far too long to connect my driven mentality, an overactive lifestyle and my continued decline in health. While I wasn't preemptive in my efforts, you can be. That's why this book makes the connection evident within the first few chapters. You'll see how your past lifestyle choices have contributed to your illness and why the choices you make in the future can propel you into a permanent state of well-being. You'll learn why you make the decisions you do and how to make better ones moving forward.

Once I realized the error of my ways, I started focusing on making better decisions for myself, ones that would prevent my lupus from flaring up. I knew if I was healthier, I'd be more mobile and have more energy. I would enjoy life like I used to. I could spend more quality time with friends, enjoy evenings out with my husband, and be the spunky, happy wife, sister, friend and daughter I once was.

Taking ownership of my life no longer seemed futile. It seemed like I could actually improve my life with lupus, if I just chose to do so. I could actually start living well, despite lupus.

During the next two years, I downshifted almost every aspect of my life. I quit my job and made it my number one priority to get myself back in good health. I cancelled vacations, passed on social engagements, and incorporated a 2-hour nap into my daily routine. Some days, the decision to live well seemed just as difficult as the suffering I had already experienced. But in most cases, it proved to be the greatest decision I had ever made.

I learned all I could about the disease. I attempted to understand its patterns and adjust to its needs, making changes and sacrifices along the way. My life was different, for sure. But no doubt, it was better. After all, I was living well. Before, I was merely surviving.

Ever so slowly, the pain, swelling, and fatigue began to subside. My failing organs and deteriorating spirit, both of which I thought were permanent fixtures in my life, started to heal. Hopelessness, despair and anxiety were replaced with confidence, happiness, and serenity. I had been trying so hard to extricate the disease from my life, I had failed to consider the positive effect of incorporating (and accepting) it as part my life's master plan. I began to see just how good my life with lupus could be. **And so can you.**

WHY THIS BOOK?

When you were diagnosed with lupus, you may have found what you thought was a sufficient amount of literature on the subject. Many books, which you probably still own and reference today (as do I), feature explicit facts about what you could expect: details about the diagnosis, the tests, and the symptoms. They touch on the different courses of treatment you might encounter, and in very unspecific terms, how you might feel about being diagnosed.

But even though you know what to anticipate from the disease, you still don't know how to cope with it. You struggle with the emotional and physical challenges on a daily basis, specifically because the limitations your body experiences conflict with the resolve your mind is manufacturing. You have an overwhelming desire to push through your pain and fight the disease without surrendering. But your efforts aren't successful. The physical symptoms are too powerful, too oppressive, and too limiting.

As a result, feelings of frustration and desperation flood your body. You can do nothing to drive those unsettling emotions away. For the first time, you feel paralyzed. You're unable to exert control over the sudden turn your life has taken. Vulnerable and violated, you begin to question your identity: who am I, what am I capable of, and what is my value to the world now that I have lupus? Your sense of self is being threatened, and you hate the way that makes you feel.

You need a proven method for overcoming the challenges you face with lupus. It's of no help to have a broad, generic understanding that swollen joints might lead to feelings of frustration. You want to know why you experience these emotions and what you can do to prevent them. You want someone to tell you that life with lupus can improve, and you need them to show you the precise way to do it.

You have never found a step-by-step approach for dealing with your illness that works, until now. In *Despite Lupus*, you'll be guided through the steps you need to take to obtain the emotional and physical wellness you deserve. There is no cure for lupus, but there is a way to live well, despite it. You could spend years trying to figure out how to do this. Or you could take advantage of the knowledge, experience and guidance presented in this book. You could learn to start living well today.

Many of the steps involved in living well are challenging. Most involve patience, effort and keen self-awareness-attributes that don't come easy to any of us. Therefore, this book contains the advice and wisdom you need during your greatest struggles with lupus. Included are tips on tackling the mental and physical limitations brought on by the disease; insight into dealing with your doctors, co-workers, or concerned friends and family members; and tricks to managing your test results, prescriptions, and myriad symptoms. In this book, I draw from a collection of valuable discussions from lupus support group meetings, inspirational and thought-provoking books and magazines, and first-hand experiences from people suffering from lupus just like you. You'll find a comprehensive and enlightening take on successfully managing a life with lupus like you've never found before. In picking up this book, you've taken your first steps toward living well, despite lupus!

A HEALTHY DEFINITION

Take a moment to think about what it means for you to "live well with lupus." Currently, your definition of "living well with lupus" may look something like this: a strong identity at work, being in control of your life, and never having to ask for help. You might assume that a high-achieving personality and an invincible attitude go along with it. You're holding fast to your definition because you're convinced that an allegiance to this way of life is paramount for triumph over the disease. But while your steadfastness never wavers, your health does. If you haven't already, you're going to be forced to re-evaluate "living well", or stop living entirely. Should you choose to follow the steps outlined in *Despite Lupus*, you'll uncover something you never thought existed: life after lupus, only better. Although it may be a slower, more accommodating lifestyle, it will be a life that is physically, mentally, and emotionally pain-free. You'll no longer worry that your joints will swell up without warning. You won't be sick and stuck in bed for days. The hair you've lost will begin to grow back, and if it doesn't, you'll be able to accept that fact with grace and dignity. Your medications will start working when and how they are supposed to, but if they do not, you'll know why. You'll no longer feel compelled to prove yourself at home or in the workplace. Instead, you'll proudly strive toward that which really matters – a long, fulfilling life that can be shared with those you love for years to come. Living well will suddenly mean enjoying life, not dreading it.

Your gauges of success will become mobility, health, and wellness. Getting down on the floor to play with your kids, holding a newborn baby with confidence, or wrapping your arms around a loved one without wincing will become markers for a successful day's work. You'll regain your abilities to think quickly and act confidently, aspects which have unfortunately fallen by the wayside during your illness. You'll be thrilled to have them back.

There won't be a life's ambition that you sidestep or are forced to avoid. The world will be at your fingertips, and you'll feel as though you've regained a life you thought was lost forever. You'll be living well and loving every moment of it.

THE STEPS TO LIVING WELL

Deciding to live well, despite lupus involves the following eight steps, each of which will be explored in detail over the course of this book. In each chapter, you'll be guided through the intricacies of each phase of your journey. You'll learn from detailed, first-hand accounts of the familiar struggle with (and subsequent triumph over) various emotional and physical aspects of the disease. You'll find specific examples and easy-to-follow exercises that enable you to successfully navigate your own way to wellness.

Here is what you can expect from the stepping stones sprinkled along the path to living well:

STEP 1 – Choose Well: Since your diagnosis, you've been fighting life instead of living it. Realize you deserve better, and choose to do something about it.

STEP 2 – Chronic Control: Find outlets for the loss of control you've experienced due to the effects of living with a chronic illness. Incorporate order, method, routine and ritual into your daily life.

STEP 3 – Look Within: Understand that the choice to live well can, indeed, be a challenging one. Look within yourself to capitalize on your strengths and make them work to your advantage.

STEP 4 – Listen Up, Doc: Learn how to best utilize your doctor as a resource, capitalizing on his/her best attributes and meshing them with yours.

STEP 5 – Communicate Wisely: Develop a genuine understanding of the role those around you play in your life with lupus. Acknowledge the benefits of involving others, and learn how to enable them to help you begin to live well.

STEP 6 – Ask for and Accept Help: Discover the benefits of asking for help, starting with easy adjustments made in your daily routine. The changes you voluntarily make today will allow you to maintain your healthy outlook for the foreseeable future.

STEP 7 – Let Go for Good: Learn to re-evaluate your goals, expectations, and sources of guilt in order to regain control of the productive and meaningful life you're meant to have.

STEP 8 – Life after Lupus: Let your new and improved perspective on life bring you a better understanding of yourself, your health and your intended happiness. Appreciate the person you've become, despite lupus, but also because of it.

Let this book guide you in your choice to start living well, and may it allow you to uncover your true happiness and potential, despite lupus.

CHAPTER 1:
CHOOSE WELL

The reality of life with lupus

Glancing at the clock beside my bed, the reality of the situation begins to sink in. It's three-thirty in the morning. I've been awake for almost two hours, and the excruciating pain and swelling throughout my body has yet to subside. My shoulders are throbbing, my hips ache, my knees and elbows are bulbous and sore to the touch. My hands are swollen into fat, deformed fists, and my normally thin, bony fingers are puffy and pounding. Exhausted, frustrated, and in pain, I contemplate my next move, knowing from experience that the hurt I'm feeling tonight isn't going to magically disappear anytime soon.

When I first awoke to the pain hours ago, I tried ignoring it, hoping to fall back asleep before it grew worse. That being futile, I maneuvered my hands, elbows and shoulders into countless positions, trying to alleviate the concentrated, burning ache felt at every point that made contact with the mattress. No arrangement of body parts seemed to help as the pain continued to resonate throughout my body. Next, I flooded my mind with positive thoughts, envisioning myself as a model of strength, resilience, and determination. I imagined healthy antibodies swiftly gobbling up the pain that invaded my body. I envisioned the pain pellets resignedly detaching themselves from my joints. I conjured up the image of pain being channeled out of my body, shooting out from my fingertips like rays of light, never to be felt again.

Unfortunately, the treacherous pain I vividly imagined vacating my body doesn't leave. Not tonight. Not any night. I lie there, wondering when I'll start accepting the fact that the pain of a chronic, debilitating disease like lupus is extremely real and very present, even if I try convincing myself that it's not.

No time to dwell on my bouts of denial now; I know I've endured enough pain and suffering for one night. I've reached my personal threshold of pain resistance, and that next dose of medication is still too many hours away to wait it out. I can't risk taking it early; I've learned the hard way that I just pay for it later. Better that I resort to my next line of defense while it's readily available: a scalding hot shower to temporarily numb the pain. Despite the agony of moving my tender, inflamed body from the bed to the bathroom, or the dry, chapped and discolored skin that forms from the harsh, hot water, the desire to deaden the pain makes it worth the attempt.

I hobble into the bathroom where I encounter my nemesis: the ancient, heavy, hot water spigot that sticks as it turns. The bones in my fingers, hands and wrists already feel like they've been crushed to bits, so the idea of wrapping them around the valve and forcing my wrist to turn makes me sick to my stomach. I know it's the only thing standing in the way of relief, however, so I clench my jaw and turn as the pain shoots up into my shoulders and back. It feels as if I've just severed my wrist from my arm, but as the scorching water rushes over me, and my body starts to turn red, speckled and numb, I know it was worth the agony.

All too soon, the water begins to run cold. I turn off the faucet and lightly dab myself dry with a towel; I can't risk awakening the aching joints I just spent fifteen minutes lulling to sleep. I crawl back into bed, hair sopping wet with a towel loosely wrapped around my body. I relish the dull, paralyzed feeling I'm experiencing from head to toe, knowing that all too soon it will be gone, replaced by familiar, raw, agonizing pain.

As I awake hours later to the alarm, I know my efforts to stave off my nighttime pain have been a success. I take my morning pills immediately, with crackers and water I perpetually keep by my bedside. I then lie awake for almost an hour while the medicine begins to reduce the swelling and ease my pain. Venturing out of bed before the pills take effect is fruitless, so I wait as my swollen, sore joints slowly return to a semi-normal state. I take my temperature, too, determining that yet again I have a fever. *That makes every day this week, with no break in sight.*

Although it's inevitable, I dread starting my morning routine. Not because I'm tired, or reluctant to begin my day, but because it reminds me of how incapable, helpless and vulnerable I've become. The simplest things, like shampooing my hair, gripping a toothbrush, or buttoning a shirt, seem like truly insurmountable tasks. Each one takes energy, courage and strength to tackle, none of which I possess any longer. A large dose of positive thinking, intense concentration and flat-out denial get me through the necessary steps, but I don't like it. In fact, I'm beginning to resent it.

In my effort to look presentable, I have found ways to work around many of the sticking points. I've eliminated any toiletries that require a screw off top or excess pressure to open. I avoid my hairdryer entirely, choose clothes free of buttons and zippers, and wear slip-on bandeau bras (no clasps or caustic under wires) to alleviate the hassle. Still incapable of grasping much of anything, I've learned to wedge the tube of toothpaste against the wall to squeeze out the amount I need, and I pin my arm against the towel rack to temper the shaking (from the medication) while I apply a couple swipes of makeup. It's nothing fancy, just enough to give my face some color.

On the surface, I'm proud of myself for muddling through and making the necessary accommodations to my routine. It takes a lot of guts to push through the pain and awkwardness each morning. If I'm truly honest with myself, though, I hate making concessions. I'm sick of putting my hair in a loose ponytail because I'm too weak to brush it through. I'm annoyed that I skip breakfast every day because maneuvering the cereal box or putting a bagel in the toaster is too taxing. I'm fed up with the pain of buckling a seatbelt, straining to punch the teeny numbers on my cell phone, or struggling to pull up my pants when I go to the bathroom. Sometimes I just don't know how much more torment, disappointment, or embarrassment my mind or body can endure.

These thoughts run through my head as I take a minute to rest on the chair beside my bed before starting off to work. My husband Johnny is still asleep, the alarm set to go off in another 20 minutes. Tears start to well up as I watch him sleeping soundly, without any difficulty or agitation, without an ache or pain. Although I make no effort to arouse him from sleep, I secretly wish that he would open his eyes, see the hurt shrouding my face, and come to my aid. *But what could he really do?* He isn't capable of ridding my body of the all-encompassing pain I feel inside and out. He isn't hiding a magic wand somewhere that can mysteriously whisk away my suffering. No, he can't make the pain stop. But maybe he could make *me* stop.

He'd take one look at my pitiful, forlorn face, and put me back into bed. He'd tell me I was crazy for going to work with a fever and with joint pain so severe I can hardly walk. He would advise against driving since I can't grip the steering wheel, and he'd assure me that if I felt as crummy as I do, my boss wouldn't want me in the office either. He'd even make the call to the office for me. I imagine that he would say all of these things, and that I would listen to him. But he doesn't, and I wouldn't.

As I silently contemplate this notion, a quiet dispute between my mind and body begins to take shape. Though I'm emotionally charged, this brief period of reflection has left me physically paralyzed. I tell myself to stand up and leave for work, but I can't bring myself to pull my knees out from under me. I remind myself that conceding to the pain is weak and desperate, but I struggle to see my body making it through the day. I want to be tough and resilient, but my miserable, useless body screams debility and helplessness. Here I am, torn between perseverance and reluctance, wrestling with the incongruence of strength of mind and fragility of the body. I want so badly to crawl back into bed and hide, but I know if I do, feelings of guilt, defeat, and despair will overcome me. It's as if determination and will power are the only personal effects I have left. If those are stripped away, nothing will remain. I've already shed enough of myself for one lifetime: my hair, my mobility, my lifestyle. I can't give away my sole sources of pride and dignity. No one should ask me to do that. In fact, I won't let them.

Building on my momentum, the uncertainty of what lies ahead springs to mind. *Will it just be more of the same, or will I feel even worse tomorrow?* Per my doctor's orders, I alternate doses of steroids from day to day, and today is as high as it gets. I better take advantage of it while I can. I remember I have a work project due at the end of the week that needs attention, and my team is counting on me to come in. I rationalize that it's more hassle to offload my responsibilities than it is to just go in and push through the day. After all, my strengths have always been tenacity, execution and resolution. I don't give up in the face of adversity. I hang in there and fight the good fight. It takes serious staying power to tackle the daily challenges of life, and I've not run out of gas yet. This day certainly isn't going to be the first.

Resolute in my decision to press on, I quietly get up from my chair and wipe the tears from my eyes. I straighten my ponytail, smooth my elastic-waist pants, and make way for the door. Glancing back at Johnny sleeping soundly, I convince myself that he wouldn't want me to wake him up anyway. Lying to myself has become another one of my strengths.

In the car, I struggle with the door, the keys and even the seat belt, all which require more strength and dexterity than I have anymore. I used to berate myself for grappling with these simple tasks; *at 26 years old, I should at least be able to buckle a freaking safety belt.* The fight has become such a regular occurrence, though, I've resigned myself to find a strategic way to deal with it. I've learned to contort and maneuver my body in ways that eliminate as much wrist flicking and twisting as possible. To get the keys in the ignition, I lean to the right, bending at the waist so that I'm practically lying on my side in the passenger seat. From here, I can insert the key into the ignition without twisting my wrist, and I have more leverage when I have to turn it to start the car. This motion (the key turning) is one of the most painful tasks I'll face all day, and I brace myself for the lightning bolt of pain. As I turn, the pain shoots through my arm, but at least the car is running. I perform a similar move with the seat belt, twisting at the waist to face the back of the seat. There, I can pull the seatbelt straight toward my body, disturbing my shoulder and elbow as little as possible. Clicking the belt in place is tough, but I do the movements in quick succession. Just like ripping off a band-aid, the faster I do it, the less it seems to hurt. The joints in my upper extremities throb as I pull out of the driveway, but I fight back another round of tears. On a day like today, when the pain is terrible and limiting, albeit not completely immobilizing, I know I'm going to have to be strong.

Once I've resigned myself to enduring the pain, no matter how bad it gets, I feel compelled to make the most of the available mobility that I have. I know that the medication will be in full effect once I get to work, and from there, I'll have three to four hours to be as productive as possible. I do more than I should, extending those hours of productivity way past my limit. I exert more energy than I have stored up, and finish the day depleted and sicker than I started. It's just so hard to fight the urge to catch up; I take what I can get when I can get it. *How else would anything get done?*

As predicted, I return home that evening, overcome and trembling with pain throughout my body. I shuffle into the house as if my knees and legs are weighed down with chains and my fingers and hands pulsate from the strain of writing, typing and driving over the course of the day. I look as though I've aged a thousand years: dark circles surround my empty, distant eyes; drawn and hollow cheeks; lips that are pale and sickly. The moment I walk in the door, Johnny can tell that I'm ready to collapse. He offers to make something for dinner, insisting that I eat before I head up to bed. I agree to some toast, and afterward, he ushers me upstairs where he assists in my nightly routine. I can't lift my arms past my head at this point, so he undresses me, puts me in my pajamas, and tucks me into bed. While I lie there in pain, Johnny massages my head and assures me that I'm bound to feel better tomorrow. He doesn't chastise me for working too late; he knows I'm in too much pain to engage in conversation, much less accept admonishment. That's not really his style anyway. We're both new to life with a chronic illness, neither of us sure of what to expect or how bad it should be. He just curls up close to me and settles in until I fall asleep, knowing that what I need more than anything right now is a supportive, loving hand to hold.

As my eyes grow heavy, a thought flickers through my head, refusing to fall away. For the past twelve hours, I've endured unspeakable pain and misery, acting as though life under those conditions is tolerable, expected or even customary. I've fooled myself into thinking that every aching step and each distressed movement I've made is part of my "conditioning", making me stronger and more resilient for the long run. But lying in bed, I don't feel stronger or more resilient. And I feel anything but normal. I search myself for a reminder of the woman I used to be: typical, healthy, young; full of energy and bursting with enthusiasm for life. When I find nothing, I become desperate to restore that feeling of normalcy. I want to prove to myself that my life has turned out just the way I'd always hoped, even if I have to pretend. Tears welling up for the third time today, I muster up the energy to ask Johnny if he wants to make love to me. Physically I'm incapable, but mentally, I want to believe that I am not. He turns to look at me. He tells me that lying there holding my hand is the only thing he wants to do; that right now, he loves me more than anything in the whole world. He promises to stay with me until I've fallen asleep, but before he's barely finished his sentence, I already have.

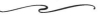

Unfortunately, I didn't realize until years later how skewed my daily thought processes had become. Day after day, I was faced with the decision of how far to push my body, and each day, I decided in error. As I struggled to keep my life moving forward, grasping for instances where I could exert control over my disease, I grew weaker and more vulnerable. Lupus began to prey on my susceptibility, striking just as aggressively as I resisted its threats. In fact, the more I ignored my body's cry for help, the more surreptitiously and mercilessly the disease attacked. Lupus was always one step ahead of me, inundating me with a never-ending supply of symptoms and side-effects. My body began to succumb to the onslaught and I suffered one disease complication after another. All signs pointed toward defeat, but I didn't know how to surrender gracefully. With no indication that life would or could get any better, I just kept fighting to hold on to the little sliver of life I still had. I assumed my battle against lupus was my cross to bear; I would just have to fight harder and harder each day to stay the course. Giving in would allow lupus to turn my world upside down, altering my life into something unfamiliar, unrecognizable, and unbearable. I was oblivious to the fact that it already was.

Perhaps you're in the midst of fighting an uphill battle against pain and suffering just as I was. Feelings of helplessness and vulnerability have taken root, and you've lost sight of any sign of health or wellness. Your objective is no longer to recover from lupus; now you're just struggling to survive. You're accustomed to operating under conditions of endless fatigue, agony, and sickliness for weeks, maybe months at a time. In fact, you no longer remember what it was like to function without them. Gone, too, are any remnants of strength, agility, and youthfulness that you once possessed. You yearn for your old self – the one that could run and jump, laugh and enjoy life with no strings attached. You want to be effective at work and valuable at home, just like you used to be. You want to feel vibrant and alive, stripped of the aches and pains brought on by lupus. Your body has been torn apart and you just want the pillaging to stop.

Perhaps you can think of nothing else but lupus. You're preoccupied with the disease, simply because it affects every single part of your life. You can't make a move without considering whether or not you'll be in pain, and that's exhausting in and of itself. Lupus hinders your ability to sleep, eat, work and play, but it also affects even the most mundane activities, like opening the mail or petting the dog. Everything has a consequence; you just have to decide from one day to the next day how much agony you're willing to endure.

Beyond the physical intrusion, you don't like the emotional commotion that you experience either. Maybe you suffer from clinical depression or like me, you're just more withdrawn, disheartened by the terrible turn your life has taken. A friend recently pointed out that the feeling of envy is actually a sadness that you experience. And when you've been stripped of your ability to function normally, how can you not be envious of what you used to be able to do? Perhaps you're even jealous of what others are still capable of doing, in spite of your own limitations. I know my sadness, while not life-threatening, was spirit-breaking. My spirit, up to that point, had always been my trademark. My spark, my positive attitude and my upbeat personality were the attributes that made me special. But each had slowly been extinguished, smothered by days of pain, suffering and insurmountable circumstances. I'd been stripped of my uniqueness and maybe you feel that you have been, too.

After months, perhaps years of pain, you begin to question your mortality. How much suffering can your body withstand? Is there going to be a point where your body just wakes up and says, **"THANKS, BUT NO THANKS!"?** I entertained the idea that my body might not hold out much longer; at 28 years old, that was a pretty miserable thought.

It's not that you want to die, although sometimes it seems preferable to the pain you're enduring. Usually, you try everything to defy the deterioration. You're determined to take on life at superhuman speed in order to evade the inevitable. You're convinced that if your body does decide to call it quits, you'll have made the most of the time you had. Thinking back, it's easy to see how irrational this perspective is. To be more concerned about feeling "accomplished" than prolonging your life is a twisted, confused perspective. But when you're living it, it seems like the only chance you have.

In this book, you will learn how to begin living well, starting right now. There's a fulfilling life out there for you to lead, despite your disease. This is the path that will get you there. To start you along the road to wellness, this first chapter will help you:

→Realize that you've already sacrificed enough
→Renew the sense of hope you've lost
→Feel empowered to make the challenging, yet fulfilling decisions ahead of you

Confronting your fears & recognizing your choices

I wish I could say that I woke up one morning, realized that I was being robbed of everything that was important to me, and made an immediate change for the better. I wish it had been that easy. In fact, I can't tell you the exact moment when I wised up, but I can tell you why I did. I realized I had a choice to make. It was a make it or break it decision, one that was a matter of life and death. Should I continue killing myself in an effort to keep my life "on track", or shed the pride, egotism, and stubbornness compelling me to do so in order to regain a life worth living? Somehow, from beyond the sea of despair I'd fallen into, I began to see that the latter had some very enticing benefits. I went further, asking myself the following:

→ Was I strong enough to relinquish the power I was frantically trying to hold on to?

→ Was I capable of valuing myself more than I value what I do or what I can accomplish?

→ Was I willing to revaluate my life in order to start the process of healing and understanding?

→ Do I value myself enough to try to accomplish any of the above?

The answer to all of those questions was and still is a resounding YES. Of course I'm worth it, and so are you.

> **"** *The question is not whether we will die but how we will live.* [1]

Making the choice to live well with lupus is a major undertaking, and I don't assume it can be made overnight. I do know that it's possible. I have very few regrets in life, but it pains me to reflect on the time I spent selfishly and ignorantly battling lupus. You don't have to spend one more moment making the same mistakes I did. You can learn from my experience, and start living well right now.

What if you're not ready or willing to accept that life with a chronic illness requires change? What if you don't want to adapt to the limitations or boundaries of the disease? Maybe you haven't yet grasped the idea that life after lupus is going to be different, despite your resolve to keep it the same. All I can say is that I know how you feel, because I felt the same way.

What if I asked you to identify and define what it is that you're really holding onto? As victims of lupus, we know all too well how customary the rigors of the disease become, so much so that we forget how abnormal it is to be in pain for the majority of any given day. We take for granted the workarounds we've created to make our lives tolerable. We've gone to great lengths to keep our symptoms under control, but are we helping or hindering ourselves? Are we attempting to heal, or are we enabling the disease to move stealthfully about its work? For example, I used to run my hands under scalding, hot water any chance I could get – at work, at home, even while visiting friends or family. In fact, I'd never volunteered to wash more dishes than I did during my worst bouts with lupus. It was one of the only ways I could find instant relief from my aching, throbbing fingers. But why didn't I take issue with the fact that I couldn't go more than an hour, if not less, without going in search of a hot water spigot to get my "fix"? Wasn't that compulsion something to be concerned with?

How about my fixation on becoming pregnant, despite my constant flares and crippling pain? I'd caught wind of the idea that, during pregnancy, one's symptoms *could temporarily* subside. Upon hearing that possibility, I deduced that it was a viable option for fending off the pain regardless of the potential risks to me and the baby, or my husband's final reluctance to participate in such a ridiculous venture. I know now that it was a selfish, dangerous and irresponsible plan, but I was desperate, and I bet you are, too. It seems worth the risk to your prevent life from being disrupted or derailed. But how great is life at this point anyway? What's so super about losing your hair, waking up and going to bed writhing in pain or taking a dozen pills to still run the risk of feeling crummy? Who really thinks that's such a great way to live?

> " *[We] behave as we do out of long established habit. To change requires more than new knowledge. There must also be an emotional commitment. Frustration, anger, discouragement, anxiety, even despair … can cause people to reexamine their lives. The hope of resolving these emotions constitutes primary incentive for change.*[2]

If your current path has led you this far astray, what do you have to lose from exploring another option? In fact, what's so compelling about *not* disrupting the life you have? If the things that are most important to you have already fallen by the wayside, why not make an about face, regain your stride, and pick up the pieces you've left behind? Don't let pride and determination get in the way. Coupled with denial, ignorance and defiance, you're only headed for more trouble than you are already in. Make the decision to start living well; choose to start today. Don't wait until tomorrow.

The power of change

When I think back to the reasons I decided to write this book, one thing becomes clear. I did not consider writing it on a day when my joints were swollen to double their normal size or the pain was so excruciating I couldn't lift a glass to my lips. Those days gave me the background I needed to write the manuscript, but the impetus for the book came during days when I felt really good, and my lupus symptoms mysteriously disappeared. It was on those high-quality days when I was reminded how wonderful life can be. I realized I was still capable of feeling normal, still competent enough to hope and blessed enough to believe. That's why I wrote this book – to celebrate moments like those and to remind others that it's still possible to live well, despite lupus.

When I did struggle to believe that my health would improve, I turned to my mom for support. Her encouragement was lifesaving, and I couldn't have survived my worst flares without her. It was during one of those flares that she shared the following phrase with me, one that I've repeated and shared many times.

> ❝ *If He takes you to it,*
> *He'll take you through it.*[3]

Regardless of your religious or spiritual orientation, a statement like this has to give you hope, consolation and encouragement. Believing that you have the stuff to make it through might be enough to get you there, but coupled with the notion that someone else is **helping you every step of the way** is the greatest security blanket out there. While the unfamiliarity and insecurity of where you are today is daunting, scary and uncomfortable, imagine the strength, courage and hope that's welling up within you, just waiting to be called to duty. "Victim of a chronic illness" is probably a label you never imagined you'd have and certainly not one you ever wanted. In fact, you don't really understand how you got it in the first place. One day it wasn't applicable, the next day it was, and it happened without your consent, input or approval. But life has a way of charting its own course and surprising you from time to time with the stops along the way. It's up to you to readjust your compass and rework the travel agenda, knowing that if you stick with it, you'll reach your destination in the long run.

THE FIRST CHOICE:
imagining a better future

Imagine for a moment the thought of living well. You might have to close your eyes to do this, since it is nothing like the life you're currently living. Envision yourself doing the things you long to do, maybe things that you've not done since the day you were diagnosed. You can probably think of activities, feelings and emotions that you believed were long gone, indisputable casualties of the disease. Whatever those lost treasures are for you, perhaps strength, agility, confidence or worthiness, picture them being restored to you as if they'd never left in the first place. Imagine the opportunity to feel whole again. Imagine the possibility of looking and feeling like yourself. Imagine the awesomeness of being filled with hope.

A friend of mine was diagnosed with cancer several years ago. She was young, single and completely blindsided by the diagnosis. She spent months in and out of hospitals, undergoing various treatments like chemotherapy and a bone marrow transplant, trying to rid her body of the cancer. During that time, she kept a journal, logging her innermost thoughts, feelings and experiences that she later compiled into a book. In one entry, if not several, she describes making a list of all the things she was going to do once the cancer was gone from her body. On her list were things like running, dancing, and singing, among many others. Although she was bedridden and staring death in the face, she believed she would regain her ability to live again. She never lost sight of the possibility. She never gave up hope. Today, she is cancer free, probably off running, dancing or singing somewhere. I certainly hope she is.

> NOW MAKE YOUR OWN LIST, including everything that you want to be able to do, say and feel once you're on the road to "living well". Jot down everything you're thinking, no matter how crazy it might sound. Don't edit your list just yet; you'll have plenty of time for that later. Instead, be as open and honest with yourself as possible. Don't be shy or reluctant about putting down things of little consequence or things that you've never admitted hurt you to have lost. Now is your chance to uncover what it is that you miss the most about life right now. It's your opportunity to grieve for yourself, while laying the ground work for a hopeful future.

Another friend of mine turned me on to this idea of grieving for my old self and lost abilities. At first I thought it would be a little depressing, but I found that it was one of the most uplifting and refreshing things I'd done since being diagnosed. For once, I was comforting myself, taking stock in the things that I really missed and reassuring myself that it was okay to be sad about it. More than that, it was okay to admit it. In drafting your own list, you permit yourself to come to terms with the resentment and frustration you've been harboring, mostly against yourself. Only when you allow the emotionally protective walls you've spent years constructing fall to the ground, can you begin to take steps toward healing. And only then can the rebuilding begin.

As you peruse your list, realize that many of the items you record today may not be things you end up choosing to resume once you've set out on your journey. You may find that along the way, the items you have listed suddenly aren't of any great importance, or perhaps they never were. You will have the opportunity to retool and reevaluate your list as many times as you need to, proactively choosing what you do and how you do it, rather than simply accepting the limited choices you had when you were unwell. Decision-making requires a level of discernment, however, so be prepared to make some difficult choices. Despite the fact that you will be forced to choose between things that you feel are equally as important, you'll be the one calling the shots. You'll no longer be at the mercy of your disease, hoping and praying that she won't strike up the band at the exact time that you need or want to be doing something somewhere. If you choose wisely, you'll no longer find yourself stuck in bed on a Friday night against your will because you will have taken great care in preparing your body for that special night by going easy the few days before.

❝ *To make Sunday satisfying, Saturday has to slow down. To slow Saturday down, we have to control the weekdays. We have to force them to march slowly in a more stately manner so they won't lump up at the end.*[4]

The choices you have on the road to wellness will be endless, and certainly of more breadth and dimension than you have now. Think of the pride you'll have in making good choices over poor ones. Another friend of mine was relating to me how her three-year old had started misbehaving a bit, doing the opposite of what she was asked to do. Desperate to find the right way to reprimand her effectively, she began appealing to the little girl's sense of independence. They discussed the idea that the girl had the ability to make a good choice over a poor one every single day. Lo and behold, the little girl's behavior immediately began to improve. Good choices inspire, heal and empower. The specific choices that we will be discussing in this book will change the way you look and feel; the way you view yourself and the world around you. You'll be a changed person, a different person, a better person. You'll feel good about who you are and the possibilities before you, allowing you to become a better spouse, parent, child, co-worker, or peer. You'll reach a new level of understanding and have the opportunity to expand your horizons, growing as an individual. You'll have found the inner peace that allows you to become the person you're truly capable of becoming, and nothing less than the best.

Up until now, lupus has squashed all signs of that good life. But when you choose to have hope, you'll be able to see and believe that life can and will be manageable, fulfilling, and worth living.

> **❞** *Affliction produces endurance,*
> *and endurance, proven character,*
> *and proven character, hope, and hope*
> *does not disappoint.* [5] *(Romans 5: 3-5)*

Think back to the hardships you've encountered up to this point. Beyond the physical torment caused by joint pain, fevers, swelling, skin rashes, poor circulation, chest pain, headaches, sore throat, swollen glands, photosensitivity, heartburn, mysterious lumps and bruises, dizziness, nausea, infections, kidney, heart and lung problems, you have tolerated enormous mental trauma including: the embarrassment of hair loss, memory problems, and cloudy thinking; the inconsistent and inexplicable nature of your symptoms; the sacrificed activities, the missed little moments and forgone milestones. Consider the effort that lupus has demanded from you to attend to the never-ending doctor's visits, medical tests, and health questionnaires. (Admit it: those hospital admittance papers and new patient forms can be a major pain, especially when you're checking off every single box under "Symptoms experienced in the last three months." You even have to write in a few that they've left off the sheet, don't you?) By anyone's standards, you've done your time with hardship, and you're an expert at enduring. Now let's turn to the future. It's time to strive for more. It's time to strive to be well.

THE SECOND CHOICE:
managing the role of lupus within your new future

But setting out to drastically improve your life with lupus may make you a little nervous. In fact you're probably a little scared. What if it's really too hard? What if this path is even harder than the one you're already on?

Think of the numerous other times when you've felt unsure (or down right scared) regarding a disease-related experience. Maybe you were able to joke about it and laugh it off, regaining your footing and reassuring yourself that things would be fine. But no doubt there were also times when you had to admit that humor wasn't enough to get you through.

I remember the morning my hand swelled up to three times its size, turned bright red and began violently throbbing with pain, all within a thirty-minute time span. Johnny and I joked that we hoped it wouldn't burst before we got to the hospital, but by the time we pulled into the emergency room, we had both fallen silent. My hand had grown so large that neither of us knew for sure an explosion was out of the realm of possibility. Another example was the second time I had fluid surgically removed from my lungs. I jokingly asked the doctor if he thought I could "top" my previous tapping, not thinking that was really possible. I'd been feeling better since the last procedure, and I was confident that I had been on the road to recovery. But as the fluid was being extracted, we saw that there was actually twice as much as there was the last time. I was bewildered and stunned, practically drowning in the agony of my defeat. Still worse was one random evening after work, when the pain in my joints was so bad it was causing me to throw up. I couldn't even stand. Per a phone call to my doctor, I tried extra pain pills, but they didn't have any effect. As I rocked back in forth in the bathtub, naked, feverish and chilled, my husband and sister pouring cups of hot water over my back and shoulders, I remember concluding that I wasn't strong enough to make it through my trials with lupus. I had been mistakenly assigned to the post, and I was going to have to take leave now. God must have simply made a mistake.

Fortunately, for me, God didn't make a mistake. I withstood those instances along with many others, each time emerging as a stronger yet more humble individual.

Gone was my arrogance, my insensitivity, or my failure to appreciate the bless-ings I did have. The hope and belief that I was strong enough to accept this burden increased with each trauma I survived. Believe me, it wasn't fun, just as I'm sure your battles with lupus have been less than amusing. That's why the quest to begin living well is such a sweet, irresistible offer.

Think, too, of all of the tangible "bonuses" that you might start experiencing: the excuse not to weed the garden, the ability to take a nap now and again and not be teased for it. When you're 80 years old, what will you be able to say about your life? The fact that you'll be *around* when you're 80 years old is a feat in and of itself. But how are you going to be able to talk about your life? Will you shine with pride, hu-mility, and thankfulness, proclaiming that you actually chose years ago to conquer lupus once and for all? Will you be able to say that instead of being held back by lupus your entire life, you seized the opportunity and made it more fulfilling?

This isn't a new concept, of course. Many life altering and/or traumatic experi-ences in life lead us to this point. Whatever gets you here (divorce, family death, or in our case, illness), it's our keen ability to see past the pain, through the hard-ship, and into the light beyond that makes us the successful, accomplished people we are today. It's the stuff we do today that makes us who we are tomorrow. Years before I was diagnosed with lupus, a college friend of mine and I fervently talked of our desire to peek into the future. We were fascinated with the notion of seeing ourselves at the random, mature age of 65 years old. I think about what a catastro-phe it would have been if, at the age of 25, I'd caught a glimpse of myself a mere five years later, crippled, practically bald, and forced out of work. I would have been incredulous of the vision, not to mention distraught and panic-stricken. Even still, had I glanced at myself just one year beyond that, I would have seen a model of good health, one with short, thick hair, enjoying the freedom that comes with retirement. I would have watched a woman travel the world with her loving husband of six years, with no children in tow, but perfectly happy in doing so. At that scene, I think I might have been even more perplexed. You may not be able to see beyond today, but I contend that you don't need to. All you need to do is to make the choice today.

That choice, given a chronic, debilitating, life-threatening disease like lupus, becomes not when or if, but how. How are you going to perceive this change in lifestyle? How are you going to deal with the accommodations you're suddenly making? How are you going to view your new situation? Will you look at your new life as unfair and inconvenient, or as a second chance to get your priorities straight? Can you find satisfaction in knowing that although you have to take a nap in order to function for a full 12 hours every day, most people would pay to have a medical, bona fide excuse to rest each and every afternoon? Will you see that, although you're not working a full-time job anymore because it was too taxing and stressful, you're able to dress yourself, stand for more than three minutes, and carry your own groceries, and maybe even your own children? Do you understand that by admitting that you were helpless in the face of lupus, you have actually put yourself back in a position of control? When you identify that a disease has, in fact, taken control of your life, you have a choice to make. You can let that disease continue to rule your everyday life, or you can take steps, not to control it, but to control the role it plays. You alone hold the key to managing a life diagnosed with a chronic illness. Why not start by unlocking that first door?

> **START BY CEREMONIOUSLY** writing the name of your disease on a piece of paper, folding it up, and putting it in your pocket. Carry it around with you, reminding yourself that you've taken the first step in "pocketing" your disease. Your job now: to do everything you can to keep that disease in its place, where it can't make too much noise or take up too much space.

After all, you have to make room for all of the things you want to do, some of the things you used to do, and a world of things you might never have known you could do. Your goal: to manage the disease, along with your own expectations, and sell the rest of the world on your newfound revelation.

CHAPTER 2:
CHRONIC CONTROL
Becoming Informed, Enlightened & Engaged

Life with a chronic illness isn't easy. It takes patience, understanding, and courage. It requires that you make decisions that you might not want to make, and it necessitates changes in areas of your life that you don't want to alter. The consequences of having lupus extend to almost every aspect of your life, so it's tempting to convince yourself that the effects of your disease are too overwhelming to combat, much less overcome. You think that because you have this debilitating, overpowering illness, you no longer have any control over how healthy or happy you could be. You're at the mercy of the disease and, sadly, you believe there's nothing you can do about it. How unmotivated you must be to improve your hopeless situation!

At present, your resistance and even indifference to making life better is understandable. Nothing you've tried thus far has worked permanently, and you have little faith that your efforts will ever pay off. You decide once and for all that life will never be as good as it once was, so you stop trying to make it anything more than it is. Why continue to exhaust yourself when you'll just end up disappointed? Disappointments in life are bound to occur, you admit, but when it's your own body letting you down, refusing to bounce back the way you expect it to, the way it should, the feeling of failure is devastating. One setback after another has worn you down, and you're fed up with the compromises. You've been hampered and hindered by lupus long enough, carrying more baggage at your age than you ever thought possible. You're negative and apathetic, no longer enjoying the things you do or the people you're around. Struggling day after day, you've grown resentful and jaded. You are unwilling to work on the state of your health because no positive results ever come of it.

I remember being in this vulnerable, precarious state all too well: fighting the battle and never winning; concluding that the easiest way out is to give up on finding a way out. If you don't make the attempt, you can't be considered a failure, right? Wrong! You are more responsible for your health and well-being than ever before, and the effort you exert can and will greatly affect the outcome. Shirking this responsibility is the worst offense you can commit against yourself, and that's true whether or not you have a chronic illness. We are the gate-keepers of our own bodies and minds, the most influential executives in determining the state of our physical and mental health. We have an obligation and a responsibility to take care of ourselves, inside and out, despite the many external factors that will try and come between us and healthful decisions. What we eat, how active we are, if and when we allow stress, change and hardship to affect us are all within our command.

Clearly, the choices aren't always easy, but no one is in a better position to make the right ones than you are. You know your body better than anyone – what works, what doesn't, what helps, and what hinders. Let's take the pain caused by lupus, for example. While you may not be able to recite the scientific, root explanation using advanced, technical, medical jargon, you are well equipped to identify where you hurt, the severity of the pain, (relative to other experiences you've had) and, if you are particularly perceptive, you can probably figure out what's worsening or lessening the pain. You have the ability to determine the internal and external factors that are affecting you and your body, not to cure the disease, but to make your life better. Once you focus your efforts on eliminating (or capitalizing on) those factors which you've identified, you can personally, and drastically, improve the state of your physical and/or mental health.

Let me stress – I'm not proposing to eliminate lupus from your life; I'm proposing a way of life with lupus that is better. An integral part of the path to wellness means becoming attuned to and staying in touch with your body so that you can take an active part in pursuing a happy, healthy lifestyle, despite your disease. Even in the seemingly autocratic world of lupus, where the disease seems to dictate everything you do or feel, you have the golden opportunity to influence, participate in, and even control, the path your life takes. Brute force, as you'll learn in the next chapter, rarely works. But strategic, purposeful, insightful thoughts and actions will bring you the results you want to pursue the pain-free life you're after. Once your mind and body accept the onus of living a healthy lifestyle, the choices you make will follow, keeping you on the permanent path to wellness.

SETTLE FOR NOTHING LESS:
the need to identify the cause and effect in your life

It's obvious that we didn't ask for lupus, and goodness knows we didn't want it. While we weren't able to prevent lupus from striking, now that we have it, we have an obligation to prevent the disease from running amuck. We have the authority to determine what happens after it hits, and how hard the blows affect us. There's little benefit in placing blame or holding a grudge; rather, seize the opportunity to thwart your disease activity in a new way starting today.

Chris Carmichael, former Olympian, professional athlete, and coach to Lance Armstrong, once found himself in need of a new approach to fitness and health. In his book, "5 Essentials for a Winning Life" he shares his philosophy for achieving a healthy, balanced lifestyle, stressing the need to take a responsible, proactive approach to one's health. "Don't depend on your doctor to keep illness away. The medical establishment is a great resource," Carmichael says, "but its strength is in treating illness and injury. Prevention is primarily your responsibility."[1] If you accept that you are the star performer in determining how healthy, alive and well you can be, you will surely succeed in achieving the rewarding and fulfilling life you're after. You rarely accept mediocre results in anything else you do. Why start now?

I had a chance to realize how substandard my personal expectations had become after one particularly trying evening with lupus several years ago. Over the course of a few hours, my body had gone from functional to practically inoperable, and nothing I did seemed to stop the progression. It appeared to me that all systems were failing; one by one, my bodily functions were shutting down. Physically, I was a wreck – riddled with pain and shaking uncontrollably. I was incapable of moving my arms or legs because of the pain and every joint that could swell had. My inflamed glands and nodes were popping up where I never even knew they existed, and my nose and brow were becoming disfigured because of the swelling. My vision had grown blurry, my breathing was halted, and I could barely utter a sound. I concluded that my body was incapable of enduring the sickening constraints it had endured one day longer, and surprisingly, my mind agreed. Both physically and mentally I was resigned to losing the battle once and for all, and I found myself whispering, through tears of agony and despair, "I think I give up."

I really thought I was dying, not because of the critical nature of my symptoms, but because of the paralyzing, far-reaching pain my body was undergoing. Thankfully, with the assistance of an emergency room staff, the insistence of my rheumatologist, a morphine drip (among other drugs), and encouraging words at my hospital bedside from my husband, sister, and brother-in-law, I made it through that evening. After I'd recovered a few days later, I concluded that I needed to start preparing myself for the inevitable - the fact that I might not make it much past my 30th birthday. I didn't begin planning the actual logistics or the details of my passing, but instead I began mentally adjusting to the idea that death was closer than I thought it was.

Yet as I thought about the events prior to my emergency room visit, I realized I had done nothing to help my situation. In fact, I had done everything to exacerbate it. I had recently taken on a trying disciplinary case at work and had worked late into the night for a week preparing notes on the issue. The day of the flare, I had risen early, was stressed about finally presenting my case and skipped lunch. In the mid-afternoon, I didn't listen to my body when it started to cry out in pain. Had I the chance to replay that entire week, I would have done things differently. I would have paced myself and offloaded some of the preparation to another manager. I would have kept a check on my symptoms so that by week's end, I wouldn't have been rushed to the ER.

I began to think that if it could have been that easy to change the course of the last few days, wasn't it just as probable that I could alter the way my life transpired in the future? Could I really make life better? Of course I could. My life with lupus was still a worthwhile cause; I just needed to start acting like it was.

While you can't shed your disease, you can accept the challenge of living with it, and embrace the life you have. You were smart, successful, happy, and independent before lupus. The difference now is that you're having a hard time believing you still are. The secret to restoring faith in yourself is to focus on areas of your life where you can still make an impact. Don't waste time on aspects of life that cannot be altered, like the fact that you have lupus. Instead, concentrate on areas where you can affect change. Doing so will bring you the satisfaction, feeling of influence, and inner strength you've been craving.

❝ Grant me the serenity
To accept the things I cannot change
The courage to change the things I can
And the wisdom to know the difference.[2]

By identifying those activities that will make the most of your time and energy, you can decidedly improve your life with lupus. You'll feel accomplished, purposeful and renewed, three things that help shape a happy, healthy lifestyle. You are adequately prepared to start fine-tuning your lupus lifestyle, so let's get started.

➔ **FIRST, begin by adding a dose of order and method to your life so that you can make sense of your disease.**

➔ **SECOND, infuse ritual and routine into your approach, creating stability and constancy in your life.**

It's time for you to begin rebuilding your life with lupus, the way you want it to be, the way it should be.

Coming to terms with your disease through order and method

As a young girl, I used to love going to the supermarket. It wasn't riding in the cart or picking out my favorite cereal that was so alluring. It was the fact that, as we waited in the checkout line, I had the opportunity to organize the endless rows of candy, gum, and mints in the aisle. I loved putting everything back in its designated place, making the shelves look neat, tidy, and orderly. It drove me crazy to stare at the disorganization. I wanted to bring order to chaos, perfection to imperfection. My desire for particularity continued as I got older, blossoming into the need to have my desk compulsively neat and tidy, my clothes organized by color and type, and my preference to eat the same thing for breakfast every day of the week. I don't *have* to do these things, but they make me feel better when I do. Disorder muddles my thinking, so the more predictable and planned my life is, the better. Then I got lupus, and suddenly stability and constancy became major challenges. The symptoms alone kept me guessing, and I found it difficult to obtain a comfortable level of certainty in my life. Tired of searching for control in places where it wasn't, I settled on creating order and method where I could.

MY METHOD OF KEEPING TRACK:
the spreadsheet

About a year and a half after I was diagnosed with lupus, I found myself thoroughly and utterly lost, drowning in an overload of information and terminology about my disease. The more baffled I became by the experiences over which I had no control or understanding of, the angrier I got. I was mad because my mind couldn't grasp what my body was undergoing, and my body wasn't reacting to the circumstances the way I thought it should. I felt I was doing everything right: taking my medications, never straying from my doctor's orders, and doing my best not to let the physical and emotional limitations of the disease get me down. But, despite my best efforts, I couldn't seem to get ahead of the disease. I had a few days here and there of symptom-reprieve, times when I thought, "Okay, this must be the turning point. Now I'm really going to start feeling better." But just when I'd let optimism and a little cockiness take hold, I'd find myself back in an old crumpled state - arthritic, pained, and unhappy – the disease flaring again.

On most days, the joints throughout my body were swollen and sore, even delicate to the touch. I tried everything to ease the pain – topical creams, hot water, medication, massage – but nothing could permanently relieve it. Desperate for reprieve, I found that if I held my hands at just the right angle, my wrists curved ever so slightly, with my fingers cascading gently toward my palm, not touching or moving, I could suspend the pain for seconds, maybe even a minute. But so what if I could make that throbbing ache go away in my hands for a couple of moments? What about the rest of my body? The joints in my knees, ankles, shoulders, and hips all felt the same way, as if someone had taken them one by one and crumpled them up like a wad of paper into the tightest ball of pain and suffering possible. The hurt was exhausting, mentally and physically, and I was tired of feeling it; I was tired of thinking about it.

It was too taxing trying to keep up with all of the aspects of the disease, including the symptoms, the side-effects and the medications. It was impossible to keep everything straight. I couldn't remember whether my fevers started two days ago or two weeks ago. I didn't know which medications were working, which weren't or which drug's side-effects were worse than the intended result. I knew my menstrual cycles had stopped, but I couldn't recall when the last one had occurred. I struggled to grasp the new language I was suddenly exposed to, relying heavily on my doctors and pharmacists to translate lupus-speak for me. Although, as resources, they were invaluable, I didn't appreciate my new state of ignorance or dependency. I was accustomed to having command of a situation, and I felt gravely inadequate about not having a firm grasp on the matters of my own body. I began to feel utterly useless, and not just because I couldn't undress myself or hold a fork or spoon without wincing. I felt worthless because I thought I was incapable of doing anything that could affect or improve my situation. Exasperated, I decided to revert back to the basics, trying to exercise a little control the only way I knew how, in the form of a list.

I drew up a list of my symptoms and medications, thinking that if they were on paper, I might be able to sort them out and keep track of them in a more organized manner. At the time, I was juggling everything in my head, and it was proving to be a frustrating and ineffective practice. I fashioned my list into an actual chart, and eventually turned to the computer to create a very simple spreadsheet in Excel™ that listed my symptoms, medications, doctors, and medical tests down one side, and the numbers 1 through 31 (for every day of the month) across the top. I thought my first pass was fairly comprehensive, listing items down the side like joint pain, fevers, swelling, and nausea, as well as the names of my major prescriptions. I planned on marking an "✗" next to any symptom I experienced in the appropriate day's column, as well as a "✓" in the corresponding box every time I took a medication. I figured this would suffice. After working with it for a couple of days, however, I realized that if I was going to make this chart work for me, I was going to need to line item everything in detail: the actual dosage of medication I took, the hours I worked, my menstrual cycle, even our travel plans.

Once I got started, I couldn't stop itemizing! It took some effort to come up with all of the appropriate categories, but after a few iterations, there weren't any aspects of my life that weren't on the chart. When printed, each month took up a full page and half, each day having a designated column where I could check off how I felt or what I did. I tried keeping the chart electronically, logging on to the computer each night to fill in the appropriate boxes. Eventually, I realized laboring over the computer was too much work, since there were days when I would collapse into bed, with little time to fuss over the computer. Instead, once a month, Johnny or I would print out a clean copy of the spreadsheet, complete with the default days of the month on top and the customary symptoms listed down the side. No boxes were checked, of course. That was my job over the course of the month. I kept the chart by my bedside and filled it in by hand each evening. It might sound tedious, but I looked forward to the 30 seconds each evening where I could check off the day's appropriate boxes: *swollen joints*, check; *fever,* check; *sore throat,* check; *heartburn*, check. As the marks filled the boxes, I began to have a clear, visual account of what was going on with my disease activity. I could see how the timing and frequency of my medications correlated to my symptom activity, how severe my specific symptoms were, and how all aspects of my life (health, rest, work, travel) were inter-related. I was able to assess how I was doing from one day to the next. Most importantly, I could determine which factors were contributing to the activity of my disease[3].

Once I actively started using my spreadsheet, I was able to establish a few very concrete cause and effect relationships. For instance, my work habits and my joint pain/swelling were obviously connected. From one day to the next, I could see that when I logged extra hours at work, my joints would be swollen for the rest of the evening and for most of the following day. But, when I came home early from work or on the weekends, I had little to no swelling. In fact, realizing that my health was continuing to deteriorate the more I worked, I eventually changed my work schedule to work one day from home, and that day arbitrarily became Wednesdays. Immediately, the number of checkmarks in the symptoms column on Thursdays was reduced by almost a third. The chart didn't lie; obviously, a day with no commute and reduced level of office activity really helped temper my disease activity.

Another example: until I started keeping the chart, I struggled to find an anti-inflammatory drug that could keep my pain and swelling to a minimum both in the morning and at night. With my tracking system, I instantly saw a pattern emerge: the current non-steroidal anti-inflammatory drug ("NSAID") I was taking once a day in the morning was wearing off by about 4:00 pm each day. With this information, my doctor switched medications to an NSAID that could be taken twice a day - one in the morning and another at night - instantly making my evenings relatively pain-free.

The chart also helped me to articulate the changes I experienced from one day to the next. I had never been definitive about how I felt, particularly when my doctor asked, because the days just ran together. But with my chart as evidence, I felt empowered to confidently share my findings. I was no longer evasive or ambiguous about how much I hurt or what my symptoms were. Now, I could pinpoint when, where and how much pain I was in, positive that I wasn't imagining or confusing the days. Sharing this information with my doctor usually prompted an adjust-ment in treatment or medication, and I know he appreciated the clues. Even if no action was needed, at least a conversation about my discoveries would ensue. I would invariably learn something about lupus I hadn't known before, and I could feel vindicated that my hard tracking efforts had paid off.

All at once, I was contributing to a solution and participating like I'd never been able to before. I felt purposeful and assertive again. While I wasn't necessarily experiencing complete relief from my symptoms, life was improving, and I had something to do with it. Even if I couldn't glean anything in particular from one week's records or another, the exercise of tracking my disease activity gave me something to focus on and to be responsible for. Although menial, filling in my chart every day gave me a sense of ownership that I hadn't yet been able to find in the tumultuous world of a chronic illness. Now, I could visually account for the reasons why I felt good yesterday but not today, rather than guess at what I'd done to make it better or worse. I was able to pinpoint allergies to medications and food, ill-reactions to blood tests and inoculations, and even identify the adverse effects that my lifestyle was having on lupus.

Of course, some discoveries were easier to cope with than others. Most of the life-style changes took a little getting used to, and they didn't just solve themselves. It took will-power and a lot of compromise, but I knew the changes were for the better. For instance, based upon the multitude of side-effects I suffered after tak-ing weekend vacations, Johnny and I re-evaluated our travel plans, cutting our travel plans in half, and spreading out our trips so that they didn't fall close to one another. We had to reschedule some trips and cancel others altogether, but we both knew it was the right thing to do. I also reconsidered our social calendar to coordinate it with my charted naptimes; changed my diet; altered (or eliminated) days I exercised; and rescheduled appointments to coincide with the days I knew I'd feel the best, just to name a few. Thankfully, my husband took a very active role in adjusting our lives around my limitations, and he embraced and encouraged my newfound outlet for disease management. He even came up with a name for my spreadsheet, which in turn became the title of this chapter: Chronic Control. When I needed help evaluating the cause and effect of a series of symptoms, he listened attentively. If I needed an extra push in making a logical cut-back to my overreaching schedule, he was there for support. We often consulted my chart to-gether so that we could make sense out of this baffling life with lupus.

Granted, I wasn't able to completely cure myself with my discoveries, nor were the connections I made anything that my doctor might not have eventually stumbled upon. But I didn't have to wait around for him to uncover them on his own. Instead, I could proactively discuss the effects I was experiencing at the time they occurred. If possible, my doctor would then treat me accordingly, giving me immediate relief. My accurate, visual chart of lupus was proving to be a lifesaver, and the future of my life with a chronic illness was improving.

Recognizing the benefits of the spreadsheet

I remember the first time I shared the idea of my chart with my lupus support group. I was partly embarrassed that my life was so out of sorts that I needed a silly spreadsheet to make sense of it all, but also that I was so compulsively organized that I'd created this geeky thing in the first place. Much to my surprise, though, the group loved the concept. Our group facilitator, in fact, asked me to bring in a copy of my creation to share at the next meeting. Imagine how ecstatic I was to bring in a visual aid! I personally had experienced a great deal of comfort, relief, and satisfaction by doing the exercise myself, but I had little expectation that someone else might be interested in exploring the primitive charting system I'd created.

Over the course of the next few meetings, I shared the conclusions of my charts, citing the correlation among my symptoms, activities and medications. Though some members of my group experienced similar coincidences, many had never made the concrete connections I had until they heard me talk, with authority, about the indisputable evidence the chart provided. Many found the idea of monitoring their habits enticing. They found promise in the idea that they could identify and learn about the patterns, if any, that existed within their disease. Given the erratic and unpredictable nature of lupus, everyone, it seemed, was searching for stability and constancy, just as I had been. There was an overwhelming desire to assert authority over the disease, to have some say in the progression of our symptoms. We knew life would never be exactly the same as it once was, but we craved the opportunity at least to have a better understanding of it. For the first time, the commonalities among those grappling with a chronic disease became clear to me and I realized I'd stumbled upon a tool that would satisfy some of our most basic needs. We needed to be *informed*, we wanted to be *enlightened*, and we had a desire to be *engaged*. If we could satisfy those three needs in such a way that allowed us to overcome the sense of powerlessness we felt over our chronic illness, our lives with lupus could improve. The emotional effects of being sick day after day can be the most detrimental consequences of a chronic illness, but finding a way to assert yourself, even in the midst of the worst flare, might ignite the feelings of hope and promise that you need most desperately during those bleak times of disease activity.

→ **INFORMED:** If I made a list of the medical happenings and bodily phenomena that I've experienced since I was diagnosed, it would be a million miles long! Just think of all of the new (and old) medical information that you currently juggle in your mind. Every time you turn around, there's something new, different, or unique about your body, your medications, or your disease. You need a way to keep yourself abreast of all of the data that pertains to you and your disease activity. It needs to be an easy, workable solution, something that you can contribute to and access without causing you more angst than necessary. Using pen and paper, rather than valuable brain space, you'll be relieved of the responsibility of mentally carrying around every bit of information about the daily happenings of your life with lupus. Notating your disease activity each day is easy, and from one week to the next, you'll have created a logical, accurate picture of how things are going. Some months might be covered in pen; others, hopefully most, will be relatively blank. Either way, you'll no longer have to rack your brain trying to recount everything from memory; the details and status of your health will be right there in front of you.

→ **ENLIGHTENED:** I disliked a lot of things about lupus, but most of all, I hated the inconclusiveness of the disease. I remember getting so angry every time my lips would suddenly begin to swell for no reason. Sure, there's a medical term for it[4], and yes, it can be a symptom of lupus, but it was embarrassing and painful, and I longed to know why it happened when it did. I had no false expectations of preventing it; I just wanted to uncover the secret reason it was occurring. Once I began charting my symptoms, I saw a clear connection between my diet, my exertion level, and my swellings. Almost immediately, I reduced my lip swellings by almost 100%.

Through a detailed spreadsheet, you, too, might be able to see more clearly the cause and effect between external factors you currently overlook and some of the symptoms that you experience. Not every consequence of lupus can be eliminated, but many explanations are out there for the taking. Let a logical, methodical system help you make sense of your disease, one enlightenment at a time.

→ **ENGAGED:** Tired of sitting back and just accepting the ruthlessness of lupus? You need a way to feel like you're contributing to your fight with lupus, one that restores your mental assurance and confidence. While it's difficult to determine when and where you can contribute to life with a chronic illness, charting your disease activity is a perfect way to make you feel as though you're doing something that might impact it. You'll feel engaged and participatory as you jot down the course of your disease for the day. You'll be tempted to find ways to make your life better, because you have the information at your fingertips. You might even begin to see lupus from a different perspective for once, free of emotional attachments and sensitivities. The straightforward, objective data you compile might remind you just how much of an advantage you have over your disease. You have the ability to work your way to wellness; lupus is just a bunch of checkmarks trying to stop you. Will you let it?

Making the tracking system work for you

Your tracking system can be as elaborate or simplistic as you choose. It's yours to utilize, so create something that is easy, effective and beneficial for you, not necessarily tailored for anyone else's use. I've dabbled in various methods to track my disease activity over the years, but the most helpful proved to be my spreadsheet. I have revised my chart many times, depending on the behavior and particularity of my disease at the time. During the months when lupus was most active, I had upwards of 25 rows of symptoms listed down the side of my page, and there were days when almost every one of them had a check mark. It's so clear when I look at my old charts now, as the sea of blue ink indicates how sick I was. But then I flip ahead a few months, and I notice how the checkmarks became few and far between. For those months, I congratulate myself for taking the appropriate measures to tame my disease. I was so proud the first time I fit an entire month's data onto one 8 ½" x 11" piece of paper. I had been able to eliminate from the list a slew of symptoms that I simply wasn't experiencing anymore. I eventually went from one month per page to three months per page, a personal triumph. The brevity of my chart was a direct reflection of my determination to get better.

You too will see the progress you're making as you chart. Listening to your body more intently, relaxing instead of rushing, or simply taking better care of yourself will all be evident conclusions once you start evaluating your tracking system. To that same end, if you ignore doctor's orders or continue to make poor lifestyle decisions that exacerbate your disease, you'll see those results as well. I'm confident, though, that you'll only make positive advancements in your quest. And when that happens, take a moment to pat yourself on the back (pain-free!) Remind yourself that you had everything to do with that improvement, even if you just kept a hopeful spirit.

Today, I keep a single piece of paper by my bedside, usually marking down a sentence or two each month if my body is in a slump. I have no need for checkmarks at this point; the minimal disease activity I have is manageable in my head. However, I constantly remind myself of the conclusions I once made from the chart, always aware that plenty of sleep at night and a nap in the middle of the day will minimize my "virtual" checkmarks.

Tracking system options:

If your first inclination isn't to create an extensive, involved spreadsheet, that's okay. There are many options that will allow you to track your disease activity, some more involved than others, but each allowing you the chance to stay informed, enlightened, and engaged. Below are some methods that you may use individually or in various combinations to track your own cause and effect cycles. The goal is for you to use the most efficient means to collect the most detailed data possible.

→ **CHRONIC CONTROL CHART (C3):** List the suggested categories and associated line items found below down the left side of a piece of paper, and the numbers 1 to 31 across the top to correspond with the days of the month. (Use some, all, or none of the items I've suggested. You may have entirely different concerns for your disease; create the chart so it works best for you.) Now draw lines to create a grid so that each number is in its own column, and each line item has its own row. (This can easily be created in Excel™, per the sample spreadsheet in the appendix.) Now, on a daily basis, check off the symptoms you experience, and fill in those fields which require specific, detailed information. Within the first few days, watch your chart take shape!

SUGGESTED CATEGORIES/ASSOCIATED LINE ITEMS

SYMPTOMS - *Joint Pain, Joint Swelling, Sore Throat, Swollen Glands, Neck Pain, Heartburn, Chest Pain, Fever, Hives, Stomach Cramps, Digestive Problems, Chills, Fatigue, Muscle Soreness, Hair Loss, Vomiting, Headache, Tooth Sensitivity, Ear Ache, Numbness, Skin Discoloration, Blurry Eyesight, Lightheadedness, Hot Spots, Mobility, Angioedema, Skin Breakout.*

LIFESTYLE — *Travel, Hours Worked, Hours Slept, Nap Length/Time of Day, Exercise, Overall Morning/Day/Night, Food, Alcohol.*

MEDICATIONS - *List all prescriptions you currently or intermittently take; also list OTC cold medications, pain relievers and vitamins that you take in addition to your prescriptions.*

TEST RESULTS - *CT Scan, X-Rays, Blood Work, Urinalysis, Bone Density Test, Pulmonary Function Test, Blood Pressure, Platelet Count, Ultrasound, Weight.*

DOCTORS — *List all doctors you regularly visit. I found that although my eye doctors, dentists,* *gynecologists, and podiatrists weren't originally treating me for lupus, they eventually contrib-uted to my treatment. Therefore, I included them on my chart.*

➜ **BODY OUTLINE:** Draw the outline of a body, with arms, legs, hands and toes de-picted. Each day, take a pen and mark down the spots where you experience in-stances of swelling, pain, or symptom occurrence. You can probably get away with one drawing per week – using a different color pen or pencil for each day. You'll be creating a very literal picture of how you feel over the course of the week, pro-viding a very useful tool to share.

➜ **VALUE OF THE DAY:** At the end of each day, assign a value from one to ten accord-ing to how well or ill you felt during the day, and write it down on a piece of paper. Underneath your ranking, make a few notes about what contributed to the way you felt that day, creating a log of good (or bad) influences. You can even assign mul-tiple values periodically throughout the day – listing separate values for morning, afternoon and evening, if your disease fluctuates as such.

➜ **JOURNAL:** Write down your day's experiences in journal form, as if you're tell-ing a story. Be sure to go back and reread your entries at the end of each week, circling or highlighting common occurrences or things you suspect might be contributing factors.

➜ **EXERCISE RATING:** Pick a flexibility exercise, like forming an "OK" sign with your fingers, and rank your level of pain, flexibility, and agility when performing the exercise one day to the next.

➜ **BOOK HIGHLIGHTS:** Purchase an informative, comprehensive book that details the symptoms and side-effects of your disease[5]. If you find yourself with a rela-tively new, particularly annoying or troubling symptom, look it up, highlight the sentence or section of the book that deals with it, and jot down a date or quick note about the particulars. You'll be creating a working notebook of the things you've experienced, with the explanations right there in front of you.

Let your choice of tracking system, be it formal or informal, written or memo-rized, be the beginning of a strategic shift in the way you approach life with lupus. Any effort you make to heighten the awareness you have of your body's condition will greatly increase your chances of improving life with lupus. You, too, can reach a new level of understanding and clarity by carefully crafting your own version of Chronic Control.

The routine rut

Despite the overwhelming success I experienced with my spreadsheet, sometimes I craved refuge from the oppressive, almost obsessive contemplation of lupus that I constantly carried with me. What I needed was a little downtime from my heavy thoughts; an effortless and uncomplicated way to relieve my mind of the worries I had. With my agonizing symptoms came the constant reminder of the struggle I had with lupus. I needed time to renew my strength and confidence in order to face what was ahead. No one can be expected to shoulder the burden of a chronic illness without some mental relief from time to time, and you shouldn't either. Finding a special way to unload the burdens you carry will help you get the mental respite you need.

As one additional benefit, the routine you develop may alleviate some of the physical strain you're under, even if only temporarily. Whatever routine you create, make it your own secret get-away, a pursuit that is special to you and you alone. Find a habit that you can look forward to, a proverbial place where you can rest your mind, refresh your armor, and prepare to face yet another day with a chronic illness. As we both know, your problems won't magically be solved, but your anxiety and worry over them will be diminished. The author of _Eat Pray Love_ expounds on the need for routines and rituals, even if they are our own, improvised innovations:

*❝ We do spiritual ceremonies as human
beings in order to create a safe resting
place for our most complicated feelings
of joy or trauma, so that we don't have
to haul those feelings around with us
forever, weighing us down. We all need
such places of ritual safekeeping.... You
are absolutely permitted to make up a
ceremony of your own desiring, fixing
your own broken-down emotional system
with all the do-it-yourself resourcefulness
of a generous plumber or poet.*[6]

Any activity will suffice, as long as it is: a) legal, b) safe, and c) allows you a few precious moments where you can unwind and relax, turning your thoughts toward anything but the distractive, disruptive thoughts of lupus. You want your ritual to make you feel grounded, give you stability and put you at ease. It should be one less thing for you to worry about, so if you find yourself fretting about your pending ritual, you're most likely not going to achieve the calming effect you want. Repetition may also be a consideration for you, allowing you to mindlessly embark upon your ritual, rather than taxing yourself to think too critically. For this foggy-headed Lupite, logical thought didn't come easily at times. Alternately, you may find that intellectual stimulation or, in fact, mild physical exertion, is just the thing you need to take your mind off your cares and concerns. Remember, this is your ritual, and the only requirement is that you feel good about it, before, during and after.

As for my rituals, I have several. For one, I find a great deal of comfort in sitting down to sip a cup of hot tea to soothe my aching body and warm the dark, cold corners of my mind. I relish the time it takes the water to boil in the tea kettle, the quietness of steeping the tea, and the prolonged, relaxed enjoyment I derive from slowly, but deliberately, drinking my hot, sweetened drink. I also enjoy the simplicity of my routine. So many aspects of life with lupus are difficult and foreign that it always helps to have a familiar, uncomplicated habit in which I can seek solace. From start to finish, the time it takes me to make and drink one cup of tea is typically enough for me to clear my head, compose myself, and realize that lupus is not too big for me to handle. Suffering cannot be quantified, but I'll admit there were times during my worst flares when it took three cups of tea before spiritual and emotional relief came. Depending on your mental and physical disrepair, you might find that, one day, you need an extra dose of whatever it is you choose as your ritual, while you're able to skip it the next.

A friend of mine introduced me to another one of my favorite rituals, which she calls "Dump the Day." During the worst of my days with lupus, I performed it religiously each evening. Now, I call upon it from time to time when I'm in special need of relief or renewal. Here's how it goes:

Step 1: Before you retire for the night, find a comfortable spot in your favorite chair or on your bed where you can sit for five or ten minutes without disruption.
Step 2: Sit quietly with your eyes closed, letting the thoughts of the day swirl in your head. The most troublesome events may surface more quickly, but allow all of the events from the past 12-24 hours to come into your mind.
Step 3: Slowly, let those thoughts, troubles, and anxieties trickle away, "dumping" them out of your mind.
Step 4: Continue until all the worries of the day have been eliminated from your mind, semi-permanently perhaps, but long enough for your mind, body and spirit to experience the relief they need.

Another of my friends turned me onto the "Spa- (insert your name here)" routine, where once a week, you take an extra five or ten minutes in the shower to treat your skin to an extra special experience using a special soap or body product. It may sound a little silly, but you emerge glowing from head to toe on the outside, as well as refreshed and invigorated on the inside. It's a special treat that you can look forward to without anyone even knowing!

I also find a great deal of consolation in attending mass once a week, typically on Sundays. It's an hour of time when I can share my greatest fears, my deepest thoughts, and my most complex discoveries with someone who listens without judgment. My little talks with God throughout any given day help too, but there's something profound about going to a special place (church) where I can arrive with my bundle of burdens and leave with an empty sack.

Here are some other suggestions for infusing your life with renewing routines and rituals. I warn you that taking time out for yourself can and should be addictive. Once you set aside 15 minutes a day (or an hour or two a week) to doing something that's important to you and that makes you feel better about yourself (and life in general), you'll find it hard to give up. Go ahead, you deserve it!

→ MEDITATE:

• Close your eyes and let your mind wander. I even find counting backwards or thinking of an animal for each letter of the alphabet calming. It may help to repeat a phrase or saying, such as, "May I be happy. May I be well. May I be safe. May I be peaceful and at ease."[7]

• Sit in front of a window with a picturesque view or indulge in nature for a few minutes, really watching and appreciating the largeness of the world and the smallness of you.

• Employ a pre-scripted relaxation technique, like those found in the appendix.

• Pray. Simply begin by talking to God, or if you prefer, use a prayer, such as the Serenity Prayer found earlier in the chapter.

→ READ:

• Pick up a book, even if you can read only one chapter (or a half of a chapter) at a time. Even 15 minutes can be enough to distract you from the cares of the day.

• Turn to the comic section of the newspaper. It's just long enough to keep your mind preoccupied and let your thoughts of lupus fall behind. You may get a good laugh out of it, too!

→ WRITE:

• Let your thoughts loose in journal writing. If you're inhibited, disregard proper grammar, punctuation, or vocabulary. Just write the words that come to you.

• Compose poems, rhyming or otherwise, to be shared with no one, or everyone, if you prefer. You'd be surprised how many creative writers (and artists in general) do their best work during the most catastrophic or troublesome periods of their life.

• Make a list of the following: the best part of your day, the worst part of your day, and one thing that you're looking forward to tomorrow. Some days, your favorite thing could be hiding under the covers to avoid the day, but that's okay. Maybe tomorrow, your favorite thing will be the time you took thinking of your favorite thing!

→ OTHER:

• Cook or bake a batch of something
• Start a collection of anything and take time to appreciate, count, or organize your wares
• Take a drive
• Spend time with your dog, brushing, petting or just loving.
• Exercise

Congratulations! You've made it through the beginning phase of your journey. Your willingness to consider and incorporate even a few of the suggested changes into your current routine is a tremendous step toward obtaining the healthy lifestyle you want. The next few chapters will continue to guide you through the retooling of your life with lupus, highlighting more specific lifestyle changes that can be made to ease your life with a chronic illness.

CHAPTER 3:
LOOK WITHIN

When I was introduced into the world of lupus, I repeatedly heard that the outlook I had on life with a chronic illness would determine my ability to cope with it. Gathering from books, articles, lectures, and first-hand accounts of others afflicted with the disease, I deduced that a strong, optimistic, determined approach would give me the greatest advantage over lupus, its symptoms and side-effects. And because I'm a happy, excitable person, with a big smile and a habit for describing most experiences as "the best ever", I felt comfortable in attempting this pro-active, positive strategy. I felt well-equipped to face lupus head-on, armed with an assertive and confident personality. In fact, I was convinced that I'd be spared from the terrible experiences about which I'd heard and read. The physical symptoms and side-effects would come, I knew, but they wouldn't be able to cause as much destruction because of the resilient, deflective mental armor I permanently wore. I saw myself muscling through whatever pain and fatigue came, refusing to crumble in the face of physical strain. I would be impervious to the sadness and despair that might accompany it, denying they even existed. I would find (if not create) a silver lining in my diagnosis, and I would keep a stranglehold on my emotions, making sure that I kept signs of struggle buried deep within. Others would never be able to perceive my hardship; I might even be able to forget that I had any. I would protect myself from defeat by maintaining control over lupus, never letting it keep me down or hold me back. I would maintain my invincibility, and life would remain relatively untarnished.

When you're as confident as I was, you don't shy away from adversity; you simply transform it into something more manageable. In my eagerness to control lupus, I was able to create a false sense of reality that allowed me to "overlook" the seriousness of the disease. In hindsight, I attribute my initial overzealousness to naiveté; I just didn't know what to expect from lupus. In fact, I wrote a journal entry about four weeks after I was diagnosed that said, "I'd like someone to confirm that once this flare is over, I'll be back to normal." The permanency of the disease was beyond my comprehension, and I was incapable of grasping the scope of lupus.

But after a short period of time, that innocence grew into gross oversight, ultimately jeopardizing my health. The wear and tear I put my body through while trying to stay upbeat, active, and "normal" took its toll, resulting in longer flares and a worsening of symptoms. Despite the unfortunate increase in medications, doctor's visits, and disease complications, I never connected my indomitable approach with the disease activity. I always attributed the flare to extenuating circumstances: a tough project at work, too many weekends traveling, or extra stress at home. It was always something "out of my control" that brought on the flare, never my own faulty behavior.

As my illness raged on, my ignorant, single-minded mentality to persevere only intensified. I'd heard that pregnancy could temporarily alleviate one's symptoms, and I thought having a baby might be a viable way to get my disease under control. Even though my body was incapable of handling the stress of a pregnancy, I convinced my husband that we should at least start trying. I immediately became pregnant, but miscarried at eight weeks. Instead of taking time to recover, I started up again, desperate not to let my aching, sick body get in the way of my plans for a family.

When duty called at work, I put in my time and then some, not wanting to appear weak or feeble. Sentenced to a weekend in bed after a visit to the emergency room, I made lists of the projects I would tackle once I got back on my feet. I needed to prove to myself that lupus wasn't going to emerge from this battle victorious.

Friends and family members tried to warn me of the trap I was falling into, but I wouldn't listen. It wasn't until a conversation with my dad that things started to make sense. He said to me over the phone, *"The reasons you've been able to handle your bout with lupus so well are the same reasons that make us worry about you so much."* My dad very rarely critiqued my approach to lupus, and while this was hardly criticism, it was a bit more discriminating than his usual "hang in there" comment. I took notice of what he said, and in time, I realized I was, in fact, causing my body more harm than good. I'd let optimism, determination, and strength of mind interfere with my well-being. The qualities I was relying on the most had been transformed into destructive weapons of conduct.

❝ *Our greatest strengths are our greatest weaknesses.* [1]

While your assets, skills, and talents make you the strong, unique person you are today, you have to be cautious about allowing those traits to impede your progress toward well-being. When you're healthy, you can experiment with physical boundaries and personal expectations. But when you're battling a painful, stressful, life-altering disease, pushing your limits or failing to be honest with yourself can be disastrous.

Making the distinction between healthy and damaging behavior is surprisingly difficult, especially when you've been able to successfully straddle the line between the two in the past. Being an overachiever and striving for perfection don't seem like inherently poor lifestyle choices, but insert lupus into the mix, and you have a new dynamic to consider. You must take time to reevaluate your behavior given the new set of parameters within which you are living. What tools do you need? A little objectivity, some self-awareness and willingness to change, all of which can be acquired in your quest for wellness. Of course, the pursuit of the good life cannot come at the price of no longer feeling, looking or acting like yourself. Rather, the goal is to preserve your strengths, keep your weakness to a minimum and prevent lupus from turning you into the unrecognizable person you are slowly becoming: sick, feeble, and unhappy. To do this, you must:

→ **FIRST, understand why you react to lupus the way you do**

→ **SECOND, identify those qualities that are impeding your ability to be well**

→ **THIRD, learn to refocus your efforts in a way that enhances your quest for wellness**

I can't deny that change is in order. But I can promise you that the healthy, normal lifestyle you're after is out there for the taking; you just have to dig it out from under the damaging behavior that has become your modus operandi.

The fighter instinct

The idea of taking care of yourself isn't a complicated notion. In fact, it's pretty darn straightforward. Living well means enjoying a life that is rewarding, productive and, in our case, pain-free. In other words, it's everything that your current life most likely is not. Why is it so difficult, then, to make the decision to live in a way that unequivocally benefits your mind, body and spirit? Logic, practicality, and level-headedness should keep you on track, but they don't; perhaps, because you're not listening to them.

Be honest with yourself for a minute: Do you respond to your body every time it cries out in pain or pleads for mercy? Do you delegate tasks to others when you're aching and rest when you're exhausted? Maybe you can recall the *one* time you asked for help at work, or the *day* you were completely incapacitated and someone took care of you. I'm not looking for the exceptions; I'm asking about what happens on a daily basis. See if any of these statements are true for you:

→ I voluntarily assume more responsibility at work and home, even when it causes me pain to do so.

→ I deny that an increase in over-activity usually results in an increase in symptoms.

→ I am intent on pushing through my pain and shielding others from seeing my discomfort.

→ I contend that maintaining a healthy appearance and disposition should be a priority in my life.

→ I am focused on holding on to the healthy, vibrant person I was before lupus, no matter how I do it.

→ I believe the best way to cope is by staying positive, even to the point of denial.

→ I want to be the first patient to ever defeat an illness of this caliber with sheer willpower.

→ I know that the feeling of pain has to be better than the feeling of defeat.

Maybe you never realized there was a pattern to your approach toward lupus, or perhaps you didn't know you had an "approach" at all. The slant you've taken toward your illness, exemplified by the above statements, isn't a deliberately detrimental one. Rather, you may have decided early on to fight this disease with everything you have, like I did, or perhaps, your default mechanisms just went into high gear. In either case, the lifestyle choices you're making come from within, based upon your strengths, weaknesses and instincts. You're predisposed to be a dynamic, courageous individual and it would be counterintuitive to act any other way. Who can blame you? You may not be wrong for taking on lupus full bore, but that doesn't mean there aren't severe consequences for doing so. Though your physical boundaries are very real, they are obscured by your combative instincts to fight lupus. You don't want to admit that you've reached maximum capacity, so you don't. You let your assertive behavior threaten your health, and you've convinced yourself that you can rectify the situation tomorrow, or the next day. But just like a fire that gains momentum, you keep pushing day after day, incapable of extinguishing it. In the recesses of your mind, you may know it's time to back down, but in the forefront is the desire to keep going and the instinct to win. Unfortunately, the battle you're waging isn't easily won. The obstacle you're up against is unlike anything you've ever encountered.

Scouting out the opposition

As a fighter, you're pretty comfortable taking on a challenge. You're able to identify, evaluate and resolve almost any problem. Even if the ideal solution isn't possible, you massage the situation to get the results you want.

But lupus isn't so easily "fixed," and it's not amenable to manipulation. In fact, your disease is downright inflexible. Lupus is a menace that refuses to surrender to the onslaughts of its opponent. It's as if the more coercion you use, the more resilient it becomes. Lupus returns stronger and more vicious each time you provoke it, more forceful and uncompromising than the time before. Bombard it with physical and emotional opposition? Lupus dodges the assault, finding new and different ways to abuse your body. Its means of attack are limitless, and it never relents. And forget about fair play; lupus has no boundaries and no rules. If it does, then they're bewildering and imperceptible, to the point of ridiculousness. If pushed beyond its limits, the disease will snap. Lupus will shift into destruction mode, prepared to end the fight once and for all. No mercy. No compassion. No leniency. Its only concern is to win the fight, same as you.

You and your disease are currently in a stalemate, neither willing to capitulate to the other. You're both set on being victorious. It's time to re-evaluate your strategy, starting with the qualities you've unleashed on lupus thus far. Traits of productivity, determination, optimism, and control would normally work to your benefit in a fight against your worst adversary. But in the case of a battle against lupus, they, in fact, are part of the problem. Take a moment to consider each of these qualities in relation to your illness. Discover why and how they've become liabilities and learn to redirect them so that they don't interfere with your quest for wellness. Remember, revising your game plan doesn't have to be difficult, it just has to be honest.

PROBLEMATIC TRAIT #1:
productivity

See if anyone you know fits this definition: A highly action-prone individual who is passionate, strong-willed, energetic and driven. Do you identify with the phrases "I have always been an active and busy person" or "I do not like to postpone things"?[2] I imagine you do. This is the trait that has enabled you to manage and maintain your hectic, demanding lifestyle up to this point. In a nutshell, you have a penchant for productivity.

So how are you adapting now that you've been diagnosed with lupus? I'm sure you feel restricted, since your activity level is now limited. How about the days when your symptoms let up, even in the slightest? What happens then? Let me guess: you seize the opportunity to get back on track, taking advantage of the brief reprieve to catch up on everything you've put off while you were too sick to do so. That sounds pretty action-prone and driven to me! You trick yourself into thinking that you don't have any limitations, fitting in every errand, chore, project or outing you've postponed. It's like you've been challenged to an "activity shopping spree" and you're grasping at every undertaking you can. You like the way you feel when you're "accomplishing", despite the looming pain that comes with it. Keeping busy is good for your soul, even if it's not good for your body. It makes you feel proud and purposeful to complete whatever task is at hand. When you're in task-mode, feelings of accomplishment far outweigh the bodily destruction that you're most likely leaving behind.

For me, daily to-do lists became obsessions. I became a slave to the objectives I set for myself, feeling inadequate if I left something incomplete. Tackling one endeavor after another became the only way I felt good about myself. My activity/achievement level had a direct correlation to my dignity and self-respect, a dangerous scenario for someone whose capabilities were compromised. I put way too much stock in what I could do on any given day, almost as if the items on my list had lives of their own. There's a scene in the movie "Proof" that depicts the kind of attitude I had:

PICTURE TWO SISTERS: a bossy, anal retentive controller (like me) and a laid-back, confused, scatterbrain. The type-A sister pulls out her trusty notebook and makes a point of crossing something off of her all-consuming to-do list, much to the disgust of the other one. The scattered sister asks, "Do you ever cheat and tick off something you haven't actually done yet?" The other one responds, "Well, I would only be cheating myself."[3]

I tackled my life's agenda as if it was the only shred of evidence that I was still valuable. I fed my self-image first, and worried about what my body could handle second. I don't think I could even discern what my physical or mental limitations were primarily because I didn't want to admit that I had any. Not only was my frenzied activity a race against the unpredictability of the disease, it was a distraction from the grim reality of it.

REFOCUSING YOUR PRODUCTIVITY:
giving yourself a pace lift

Perhaps you, too, have been blinded by the *"euphoria of accomplishment."*[4] Your self-image is wrapped up in what you can or cannot achieve and your self-esteem suffers when you no longer complete your objectives. In fact, you worry that you wouldn't recognize yourself without your ability to accomplish.

Alexandra Robbins, author of *The Overachievers: The Secret Lives of Driven Kids*, wrote an article for *Forbes* entitled, "Confessions of a (Recovering) Overachiever". In it, she says, "There are two kinds of overachieving: the healthy kind, when you can't stop doing what you love because you enjoy it, and the unhealthy kind, when you stack up accomplishments as if etching notches on a bedpost." [5] Have you fallen into the habit of craving notch-like accomplishments such that nothing less than the best is good enough? It isn't realistic and/or feasible to seek such perfection and efficiency when you are sacrificing your health to do it. You can't and shouldn't dismiss your desire to achieve entirely. But, you can look for alternative ways to get the accomplishment rush you need. You can still feel good about yourself without risking your health to do it.

Begin by valuing yourself, not for the things you can accomplish, but for your ability to recognize what's collectively best for your mind, body and soul. Don't berate yourself for a loss in productivity or stamina. Instead, remind yourself that, while your disease limitations force you to make decisions, with decision-making comes the advent of choice. When you're on the run and in a big hurry to get things done, you may miss a few things along the way: the fleeting opportunity to spend a few extra minutes with someone, the chance to catch a beautiful moment in nature, or the possibility to learn something new. These things would never make your to-do list, not because you didn't want them to, but because you never contemplated the choice of doing so.

Force yourself to discriminate between what you have to do, what you want to do, what you can do, and finally, what's really important for you to do on a daily basis. By managing and prioritizing your undertakings in a way that satisfies your mind, but doesn't endanger your health, you will undoubtedly find happiness. Today, I juggle more responsibilities than I ever have before, but in a healthier, responsible manner. I no longer rely on frantic, desperate activity to quench my thirst for approval. A renewed sense of self satisfies that need. I know who I am and who I want to become; I no longer look to a laundry list of items to tell me.

❝ *You cannot see your reflection in running water, only still water.*[6]

Begin your quest for wellness by giving yourself a "pace lift", using these three guidelines to start. Determine how important the feeling of accomplishment is to you personally, and then design a healthy lifestyle around it.

1) PRIORITIZE YOUR ACTIVITIES

Instead of focusing on all the things that have to get done, try eliminating the tasks that can actually wait. You'd be surprised how much easier it is to manage a list of three items versus five, even if the remaining three demand a considerable amount of time and energy. Your list won't seem as frustrating or daunting once you've eliminated "weed the garden" or "take on extra project at work" from your list, things that just don't make sense in your current state of illness. No one but you can truly judge the import of what needs to get done, but that's the beauty of it. You can take control by choosing one task over another, opting to only do those things that will bring you the greatest degree of satisfaction and benefit.

2) ELIMINATE "SHOULD"

A friend of mine from my lupus support group came up with this, and continues to share this bit of advice with new members of the group. Every time you think about something that you *should* do or that *must* happen, rethink it for a moment. Does it really have to happen or do *you* just want it to? Many things on your plate have to get done, but I'd be willing to bet the list that you deem obligatory could be cut in half if you would take a good, hard look at your "should" usage. Here's another refreshing way of looking at it:

THE LATE POPE JOHN PAUL II WAS ONCE ASKED WHAT HE DID IN HIS FREE TIME. HE RESPONDED WITH SOMETHING LIKE, "ISN'T IT ALL FREE TIME?"

When you view life in this way, it becomes clear that your frantic desperate "musts" might be energy ill-spent. Choose to do that which you enjoy, endeavors that test your intellect, creativity, or even stamina. The point isn't to exceed your limits. It's to challenge them in such a way that you find fulfilling.

3) FOCUS YOUR ENERGY ON THE PRESENT TASK

You may have heard that multi-tasking can actually be less productive than focusing on a single task. Have you ever considered the drawbacks of "multi-thinking", the tendency to think about the other things you're going to do once you finish that which you are currently doing? How many times have you tried to take a quick nap, but couldn't fall asleep because of the thoughts roaming around in your head? You toss and turn, frustrated because after 30 minutes, you still haven't fallen asleep. Your mind is a constant swirl of ideas and plans about what's to come, so you have to train yourself to focus on the task at hand. Learn to maximize the time and energy you have, especially since both of these are now limited.

The next time you nap, practice the act of relaxing rather than just lying down and closing your eyes. Remind yourself that the only objective at that very moment is to rest, and nothing else. See, hear and feel yourself resting. Imagine your mind relaxed; considering it to be on break. If you're hyper-focused on resting, your mind won't be able to wander. This goes for any activity that you find is not as productive as you'd like it to be. Whether it's a workout, a trip to the grocery, or a visit to the doctor, envision a spotlight in your mind, singling out the thing that you're doing, and focus on the task at hand. Take full advantage of the resources in front of you, and I'd be willing to bet that, soon enough, you'll be able to accomplish what you want in even less time than before!

PROBLEMATIC TRAIT #2:
determination

Even before I had a lupus diagnosis, I was determined not to let the symptoms of the disease derail my life. Two weeks before Christmas, I noticed a tightening in my chest when I breathed in or out. It was a heaviness that I couldn't easily describe, but I attributed it to indigestion or heartburn and carried on with my Christmas to-do list. With presents to wrap and cookies to bake, I didn't have time to worry about a little chest pain. *Just push through like you always do.* As I went about my errands over the next few days, my breathing became even more labored. I found myself doubling over because of the sharp, intense pain that shot through my side and back. At night, the pain would swell up in my chest, often leaving me gasping for breath. I knew something was amiss, but I resisted making a doctor's appointment. We were traveling for the holidays, and I certainly wasn't going to delay our trip. Whatever I had would have to wait for a diagnosis until we returned. I was rarely sick, and while this seemed a little out of the ordinary, I wasn't going to succumb to the pain. I just needed to strap on a little tolerance, and I'd be okay. *Who goes to the doctor for something like heartburn, anyway?*

I wish I could say that after I sought a doctor's opinion and learned that I had lupus, I readjusted my thinking. Unfortunately, my willfulness only intensified. Months after I was diagnosed, I was still trying to muscle through the pain. One evening, in particular, I refused to cancel our evening plans, despite my aching joints and overwhelming fatigue. We'd planned on meeting friends out for dinner and drinks, and I'd already canceled another outing earlier in the week. *Wasn't that enough? Couldn't lupus just beg off this once?* I was hopeful that tonight would work out and was determined to make it happen. Trying to set myself up to succeed, I'd intended on leaving work early that day, giving myself time to rest before dinner. I learned the hard way that attempting to go directly to another event from work was futile. If I took a quick nap, I'd be able to make it through an entire evening without becoming a damaged, dilapidated mess. At least I had a better shot of it, anyway.

As was consistently the case, though, I left work later than planned. I arrived home, completely exhausted and crippled from swollen, painful joints. Johnny could tell I felt terrible, but I assured him that I'd be okay after I lay down. I hobbled upstairs, collapsed into bed and fell asleep instantly. Less than an hour later,

Johnny came in and whispered that it was time to leave. Although I tried to move, I could barely lift my head to acknowledge him. I was utterly spent, wiped out from a long day and a long week. He offered to cancel our plans, *again*, but I told him to go ahead; I'd meet up with him in time for dinner. "Don't worry if you can't make it tonight," he said as he kissed me on the forehead. "Everyone will understand." I maintained that if I could just get a little more rest, I'd be able to make it for sure. He put the phone by my bed, asking that I call him before leaving. I promised to do so, but knew he would try to talk me out of coming when I did.

"I'm going to make it, Johnny. You just wait and see."
"I know you will, Sara. I know you will."

Three hours later, I woke up from a dead sleep, devastated when I saw what time it was. I'd missed drinks, dinner and the entire evening. Lupus had ripped another night out from underneath my feet. I was so frustrated that my body had become so needy and angry that I'd let myself give into it. I called Johnny to let him know I hadn't even made it out of bed. He sensed my disappointment, but assured me that I'd needed the rest. Everyone sent their well wishes, and he agreed to tell me every detail of the evening once he got home. In my opinion, it was a sorry consolation prize. The physical ailments had gotten the best of me that night, but I was determined not to let it happen again.

Even before lupus, I was the epitome of headstrong. I believed mental resolve was the key to success, so I rarely backed down from any challenge. When a situation turned bleak, that's when I began to thrive. At work, I was the cheerleader who encouraged others to push beyond their limits to get a job done and to do it well. Fueled by a driven personality, I rarely accepted "no" as an answer, even at home. When I did, I was the one initiating it. In fact, the nickname my family gave me in my early twenties was "The Godfather". Most of the time, it was very fitting. I had an agenda and planned on seeing it through, regardless of the sacrifices I had to make. Winning was always the goal.

REFOCUSING YOUR DETERMINATION:
learning to compromise

Who doesn't like getting their own way? You're a fighter and like me, you enjoy winning. Despite lupus, you're attempting to push through life as if nothing has changed. But the pieces of your life don't fit together the way they used to. Some may be damaged, others broken and still others may be missing altogether. Yet you're exhausting yourself with mindless comparisons and foolish expectations. You think if you could walk for an hour before lupus, you should be able to walk for an hour after lupus. If six hours of sleep was enough before, than six hours should suffice now. You're spending way too much energy trying to recreate your life, when you should focus on rebuilding it.

Your persistent nature has gotten you this far, but it's now getting you into trouble. Though your mind is wired to resist the limitations it's experiencing, your body isn't capable of staving them off. It's time to revise your strategy. Begin by inviting compromise into your thought process, laying the groundwork for change. Don't let your instincts drive you to just grin and bear it anymore. Instead, retool your thinking so that a little give and take becomes an acceptable means of getting what you want. How do you begin? Slowly permit yourself to make accommodations in your lifestyle where you might not normally make them. In essence, practice being a little less perfect.

> ❝ *The thing that is really hard, and really amazing, is giving up on being perfect and beginning the work of becoming yourself.*[7]

The following suggestions will help recondition your mind to view compromise (and ultimately change) not as the enemy, but as a means to a healthier, happier lifestyle.

1] EASE INTO IT

Start with a habit that, if altered, would bring you immediate relief, like the amount you sleep at night. Although you know an extra hour or two of sleep would help, you can't seem to get out of the habit of going to bed when you always have. Whatever that time is, it's too late, since you're still tired in the morning. You've tried moving your bedtime up by an hour, but something always gets in the way. You work late, the kids need help, or something in the house needs attention. Before you know it, 45 minutes have gone by and you're almost back to your old bedtime.

Perhaps a full hour is too much to ask yourself to give up right at the start. Begin, instead, with just 15 little minutes, a time commitment that is manageable, even with the evening emergencies that arise. Do this for a week or two, but don't be upset if you miss a day here or there. Just keep at it and soon enough, your bedtime will be 15 minutes earlier. Now work on gaining another 15 minutes once you have the first 15 down pat, and so on and so forth. Soon enough, you'll have shaved off that hour.

Whether it's going to bed earlier, drinking more water or getting more exercise, making incremental changes to your routine gives your body time to acclimate to the new pattern. Because we instinctively resist change, the more subtly you go about it, the more likely you are to succeed.

2) INDULGE, BUT WISELY

A friend of mine was struggling with the sacrifices that lupus was forcing her to make, like reducing her sun exposure and restricting her activity level. She had a chance meeting with another woman who had grappled with the same things, but who had come to the following conclusion: indulging every once in awhile in an activity that is deemed "off limits" is okay if you allow yourself ample time before and after to recover. This woman happened to be an avid tennis player and it was causing her more stress and anxiety to miss out on a match than to deal with the effects of playing one. Given that her body was more fragile and prone to exhaustion with lupus, she realized that if she took it easy the day before and after she played, she could enjoy her pastime and not put her health at risk. As long as you're willing to compromise, you can enjoy doing just about anything.

Keep in mind that a compromise like this one should be viewed as an indulgence, not an invitation to develop a routine. Don't let the thrill of the experience convince you otherwise. Just like eating a cookie on a diet, it's not the *one* cookie that does you in. It's getting a taste for it and wanting a second, if not a third.

In addition, be resourceful and open-minded when devising ways to enjoy yourself without jeopardizing your wellness. My in-laws recently planned a wonderful day trip to New York City for sightseeing, shopping, lunch, a Broadway show, and dinner, complete with a limousine ride to and from the city. It required about four hours of traveling each way from where I live – too much for me to tackle in a single day. I didn't want to miss the trip, but I couldn't figure out a way to go without exhausting myself and running the risk of getting sick. After brainstorming with my husband and his family, we decided that my sister-in-law and I would skip the limo ride, take a train up the morning of the show, stay overnight with family in the city and leisurely make our way back via the train the next day. The scenario couldn't have been more perfect! I would have the option to rest midday at my in-law's place, crash early, sleep in the next day and still enjoy all of the festivities. I had to compromise and skip the fancy entrance and exit into NYC, but it was worth it. Exercise a little discretion, and I think you can have your cake and eat it, too!

3) PRACTICE NOT BEING PERFECT

You just can't wake up one morning and decide to stop being organized, prepared, or driven; you actually have to work at it. Make it a game by picking one thing each day that you're going to let "slide." Maybe it's foregoing one non-urgent item in your in-box, getting take-out for dinner instead of cooking an elaborate meal or putting away the laundry tomorrow and not today. Your life won't get sidetracked one allowance at a time, and you'll grow more comfortable in the company of your own imperfection - a valuable attribute, no matter who you are.

PROBLEMATIC TRAIT #3:
optimism

Who can argue with the benefit of positive thinking? Without a doubt, it is one of the most highly touted and proven methods for dealing with the problems we encounter in everyday life and with good reason, too. A positive outlook gives you confidence to face the day ahead, eases your mind from worry and stress, and can bring you success and happiness in a way you never thought possible. I consider myself lucky, since maintaining a positive outlook on life comes naturally to me. I rarely struggle to fight negativity or pessimism because my upbeat and cheery disposition usually squelches feelings of doubt, sadness, or discontent before they take hold. I can't claim that I've never experienced unhappiness or disappointment; I just find it easier to dismiss the situation and move on to more pleasant thoughts than to dwell on the unfortunate. Perhaps I'm distancing myself from my true feelings, but that detachment has never held me back from living a life that I felt was meaningful and worthwhile. Of course, my illness and the complications that accompany it certainly tested my outlook on life, but I knew it was essential that I maintain a good attitude. I focused as little on the negatives of lupus as possible. I believed that in doing so, I could prevent them from fully manifesting. I would play up the good, overlooking the bad, even if it meant subconsciously making the situation out to be better than it was. In my mind, I was just masking the symptoms in order to help me cope with the ordeal. In reality, I suppose I was ignoring the truth.

While some might jump to label this "denial," I'm reluctant to do so. Denial, to me, implies a negative refusal to do something. I promise you, there wasn't anything negative about my approach. What I suffered from was an inability to see what was happening to me, not a refusal to do so. I was overwhelmed by the barrage of symptoms, complications, and limitations, all of which were unfamiliar and unexpected. I found myself lost in a sea of opinions, advice, and suggestions, and I struggled to make sense of them. My hopes and desires, both of which had been clear and well-defined, were suddenly blurred and uncertain. I grasped for direction. Inundated, I thought my best defense was to stay unnaturally and extraordinarily positive. I closed my eyes to the adverse effects lupus had on my life, incapable of dealing with them in a rational and logical way. I had no concept of what my body needed or suffered from anymore, and I had become as ignorant and unaware of myself as I'd ever been.

REFOCUSING YOUR OPTIMISM:
breaking the spell

At some point along your journey, you're bound to lose your objectivity, too. Given the myriad aches, pain, swellings, rashes, and fevers to which you're subjected, do you really know what "good" should feel like anymore? I'm not asking if you can describe the feeling; I want to know if you remember what it actually feels like. I bet it's been so long since you felt 100%, you no longer can imagine that exact sensation. Passage of time, conditioning, and relativity have recalibrated the measuring stick you now use to determine how much hurt is enough, and how truly sick you are. The gauge you use today can only be the pain from yesterday, but how insufferable was the pain even then? Maybe your complaints are fewer than they've been in the past, but why should functioning with *any* health complaint suddenly be acceptable? An objective assessment of your health is no longer possible because you've reduced your expectations to accommodate the changes in your functionality and appearance. The ailing, broken-down, failing body you see in the mirror somehow looks more familiar than not. It's as if "normal" has been redefined to mean "that which is bearable" and the ache in your hip or the joint pain in your hands is now customary. Your standards have been compromised. Now it's time to reconsider what "normal" should really look and feel like.

1) MAKE IT RELATIVE

Pick an unhealthy habit or activity that you currently overlook or dismiss. For instance, let's say you have the tendency to work through lunch. You know taking a break has benefits, but you've convinced yourself that it's better to just get your work done. Why? Maybe it hurts to walk all the way to the lunch room, or perhaps your illness has taken away your appetite. You've lost perspective, and that's understandable. But regain an objective point of view by asking yourself what *you* would do if you saw colleagues skipping their lunch break day after day. What would you say to them? Force yourself to come up with a few, indisputable reasons why your "colleagues" should break for lunch. Write them down and then sign your name to it. Now take yourself up on the good advice. Reread the reasons each day, if necessary. Eventually, you'll come to remember how "normal" it is to break for lunch.

Note: *You can also employ a trusted colleague to help you with this, if it's appropriate and you're comfortable doing so. If possible, ask him/her to swing by your office at lunch time once in awhile, and let him/her take part in encouraging you to treat yourself well.*

2) KEEP A JOURNAL

By keeping a journal routinely, you'll be able to create a working benchmark for yourself. You'll be able to look back and compare how you're feeling one entry to the next. Maybe you'll be pleasantly surprised at how much better you're feeling. Perhaps you'll notice that you've had the same symptoms with no sign of improvement for awhile, indicating that it's an issue you need to take up with your doctor. In either case, re-reading your entries will give you a clearer, more objective view of what and how you're feeling, which can easily be lost in the daily grind of your mind.

3) RATE THE DAY

Start by simply assigning a value from one to five each day based upon how you feel, one being the worst and five being the best. Keep a piece of paper by your bedside so that you can routinely jot down each day's "value". If you do the exercise in the morning, on the days that are three or below, remind yourself to go easy. If you do it at night, evaluate why you think that day might have been particularly good (or bad), and make a promise to yourself to replicate (or eliminate) the activities that made it so.

PROBLEMATIC TRAIT #4:

control

During the course of my first two and a half years with lupus, I made more than a dozen trips to the hospital for various out-patient surgeries, emergency room visits and invasive procedures and tests. Never once had I been held overnight, but even still, I considered myself pretty comfortable with the whole hospital routine in general. At the end of this period, I became very ill, and my rheumatologist thought it best to admit me to the hospital, due to the possibility of internal bleeding and other alarming symptoms for which he could find no explanation. Although he told me that I was being admitted, he didn't mention the concept of being held overnight. Therefore, my expectations were the same as always: to be seen, evaluated, and released over the course of the same day.

When my doctor told me later that evening over the phone that, actually, no, I would be staying overnight, I was in disbelief. As I hung up the phone in my hospital room, I burst into tears. I knew I was sick and I wanted answers, but this overnight business wasn't part of my plan. I hadn't expected nor had I chosen to stay overnight and, yet, there I was, forced into a situation over which I had no control. I felt duped, even trapped, not by my doctor, but by the disease itself. Lupus had finally ascertained control of the situation, and I hadn't prepared for that to happen. I'd always been able to rise beyond her wrath and regain command of the situation, even if only in my own twisted, optimistic mind. Not this time. I probably should have been more nervous about was wrong with my body (since I ended up being hospitalized for seven days), but the thing I remember the most about that night was the utter despair I felt as I saw my deliberate, purposeful, well-planned life falling apart before my eyes.

Never before had I felt such vulnerability or helplessness. The tears that came throughout that evening were filled with pain, resentment, and disappointment, emotions I didn't even know I had. The feeling of failure was overwhelming. I could feel the last strand of control slipping from my fingers into the hands of the disease. I was powerless, and it was the most terrible, discouraging feeling I'd ever experienced. My life had become utterly unmanageable, and I could no longer separate my life from my disease. They had become one in the same, no longer two separate compartments of my mind. Lupus was out of control, and so was I. So it was there, amongst the tears, the desperation, and the solitude, that I decided that my life with lupus needed to change. The truth is it already had.

REFOCUSING YOUR CONTROL:
loosening the reins

Understandably, we are resistant and reluctant to change, especially when we are not the ones initiating it. No one enjoys relinquishing power or having their life's agenda rewritten without their consent, including you and me.

Maintaining control over life gives you confidence, stability, and peace of mind. You feel good when you assert yourself; content and settled when life follows the path you intend. But when life is forced upon you, without your consent, as your chronic illness has been, you panic. You rush to defend yourself against the intrusion, fighting to preserve the comfort and control you've always known. Not only are you seizing the past, you're grasping at the future. You believe your plan is the only one that will lead you to your desired destination, and anything else is a ruse. If you don't push, kick and scream against the unexpected tangents of life, life itself is liable to pass you by completely.

Like a kid who's exhausted but refuses to go to bed, you convince yourself that everything fun, exciting and worthwhile will happen if you let someone else tell you what to do. If you yield, your chance to live life to the fullest will be lost. But step back for a moment and ask yourself where your controlling, stubborn behavior has led you thus far. Has it led to a life worth living or to a life of never-ending struggle, illness, and loss?

THE HARDER I PUSH, THE SICKER I GET
THE SICKER I GET, THE LESS I RESEMBLE MYSELF
THE LESS I RESEMBLE MYSELF, THE HARDER I PUSH TO
TRY AND REGAIN SOME SEMBLANCE OF WHO I USED TO BE.

Thinking you can beat lupus without compromising one iota of your life is what perpetuates the cycle, but two things can end it: your body gives out or you give up control. Unfortunately, the former can and will happen, although no one likes to admit that it's possible. We think we're invincible, but in fact, the body can only tolerate so much suffering. If pushed too far for too long, our bodily functions will slowly, but assuredly begin to fail. It's only a matter of time. However, this outcome never has to be considered, if you're able to relinquish the control you've been holding onto so desperately. In doing so, you are instantly relieved of the burden to force order, method and purpose into your life. It releases you from your futile attempts to possess a power that, perhaps, isn't yours for the taking. You no longer have to exhaust yourself keeping to a path that isn't set in stone. Where you've been merely struggling to survive, you can, at once, begin to thrive.

> ❝ *Thrive: Make steady progress; be at a high point; grow strong and healthy.* [8]

My epiphany in the hospital sparked changes in my life that I didn't think I was capable of making. It didn't happen all at once, as you'll see over the course of the book. But there are definitive stepping stones that can help transform your life into something that once again thrives. Relinquishing the control you think you need to survive is one of those first steps. Remember, your goal isn't to rule over life, it's to live it. The moment you make this transition is the moment your life with lupus becomes one worth living.

1) REALIZE IT IS NOT YOUR FAULT

Pick three areas of your life that have changed since you were diagnosed with lupus. You can probably think of dozens of examples, but right now, focus on just three. Perhaps it's your ability to walk your dog, have patience with your spouse and take on extra projects at work. Whatever three things you feel in your life have been compromised by lupus, write them down. Now, beside each of them, write, "It's not my fault." Realize that you aren't to blame for these alterations in lifestyle. They are either the direct or indirect result of being diagnosed with lupus, and you weren't in control of getting lupus. You didn't choose it; it just happened.

By no means does this excuse you from taking responsibility for your actions and dealing with the fact that you have an illness. But what it does mean is that you can no longer blame yourself or feel bad about "allowing" these changes to occur. Lupus, in addition to being chronic, systemic, and debilitating, is also life-altering. Acknowledging that life is going to be different with lupus stops you from blaming yourself for your sudden limitations (most of which are out of your control anyway). It will allow you to start dealing with the disease the best you can.

2) CONTROL THE ROLE

Imagine your life as one big theatrical performance (not too difficult, right?). You are, of course, the star of the show, and those close to you will be playing the requisite supporting roles. Now assign lupus a role in the production – that of stagehand. Lupus' job is to be as inconspicuous as possible: to stay behind the scenes, disrupt nothing, and if movement is necessary, attempt to blend in with the scenery. You give this very special, important role to your disease, not because you necessarily want it around, but because you know it's not leaving anytime soon. Acknowledging that it's a part of the play and giving it a job to handle will hopefully keep it busy and out of your way, allowing you to give your best all-time performance.

As you act out the scenes in your life, ask yourself the following: is what I'm about to do going to allow lupus to upstage me? Will my disease, who's supposed to be waiting idly behind stage, have an opportunity to run across stage, leaping and bounding and causing a scene? For example, if you work extra late, or refuse to go to the doctor, will you be encouraging lupus to crash the scene? Keep these things in mind as you go about your daily performances and allow yourself to be the center-stager you're meant to be!

3) FIND NEW WAYS TO CONTRIBUTE

Don't waste valuable time and energy trying to control areas of your life that aren't meant to be tamed. Instead, focus on finding new, yet equally effective ways of making life worthwhile. For instance, maybe you've discovered that after an hour of working diligently on a task, you find it difficult to concentrate, get bleary-eyed, and are no longer productive. It's a mystery why this happens with lupus, but somehow, your disease can't tolerate working on something too long. Don't fight the new wrinkle in your work style; instead, accommodate it. Work diligently for an hour, take a small break, and then get back to it for another hour. If you try and push yourself to work straight through for two hours, you'll end up spent and ultimately lose out on valuable productivity time. You are as valuable a resource as you've ever been; you just have to reevaluate how you can still make an impact.

Self-awareness to the rescue

Consider section one of your quest for wellness complete! The three chapters you just finished asked you to do some heavy soul-searching and make some definitive changes in the way you perceive life with lupus. The momentum you've built will only keep you going in the right direction. In the next section, we'll look at the role others play in your quest. Believe it or not, doctors, family members, friends and co-workers all play a vital role in your journey. Discover how you can learn to manage them so that they can help you manage lupus.

CHAPTER 4:
LISTEN UP, DOC!

The first impression I had of my rheumatologist ("Dr. R") when I met him more than eight years ago was that he was a little quirky. What am I saying? He still *is*! His offbeat sense of humor and sometimes abrupt style make for a unique bedside manner. Nevertheless, his thoroughness, experience, and track record have made me a lifetime devotee. When I'm sick, he cures; when I'm healthy, he works to keep me that way. Dr. R is sharp, intuitive, and relentless when it comes to solving the lupus enigma. I wouldn't have made it this far had it not been for his treatment and intervention. Thankfully, over time, his more pleasant, patient, and caring personality traits have surfaced, where they've remained in full force. Today, only his strengths shine through, and I've come to enjoy, if not look forward to, my appointments with the infamous Dr. R. It's a good thing, too, because the time I've spent with him hashing out the symptoms of my disease has been considerable. He saw me every two weeks for months before slowly ratcheting back my visits to four and then, eventually, eight weeks between appointments. There were emergency office visits, late-night and weekend crises and countless phone calls, most of which resulted in, you guessed it, more office visits.

In the beginning, I wanted education and direction, someone to lead me through the trials of lupus. He must have sensed that I was lost and bewildered in this new state of sickliness, because he responded with appropriate guidance and authority. He immediately took charge of my treatment, working closely with my other doctors, informing or consulting with them whenever necessary. He spent a great deal of time with me during my appointments, even fitting me in for emergencies. He made follow up calls to see how I was feeling between visits, making me feel important and valued, not sickly and deprived the way lupus makes you feel. He answered every question I threw at him, and those he couldn't, he researched and got back to me at my next visit. I turned to him to translate, interpret, and diagnose everything regarding my health, and he responded appropriately. As new symptoms or problems emerged, I waited patiently until I could unleash my latest lupus sufferings on Dr. R. Once I did, I felt relieved knowing that I could collaborate with someone more knowledgeable and capable than I was.

Over the years, I have unloaded every health crisis and complication on him, often in fits of desperation, frustration or incomprehension. I entrusted my life and health to this man, who without fail listened intently, acted confidently, and performed what appear to be miracles. Dr. R knows and understands more about my life with lupus than anyone else. I don't know how one can battle a chronic illness without such a formidable doctor. What a vital role he plays in my life, giving me the means to become a healthier, happier, more active individual.

With lupus, there's no medical professional you see as frequently or intensely as your primary lupus doctor (usually a rheumatologist). And, just like any other relationship, the alliance between doctor and patient must be endurable, agreeable, and effective if it is to be successful. It's a partnership, requiring two willing and able parties to share the burden and the responsibility. That means you *and* your doctor must work at the relationship, not one independent of the other.

For some time, I didn't realize that Dr. R needed my assistance in this way. I thought optimizing my treatment was his responsibility alone. He's the doctor, after all, the one with all the answers, resources, and schooling. Over time, I realized how I had underestimated the role I needed to play as a patient, both in and out of the doctor's office. For starters, instead of assuming that he automatically knew what my expectations would be as a patient, I needed to discover what they were myself. Once I figured out what aspects of my doctor's visits were most important, (*i.e.*, having a strategic medical plan of attack at the close of each visit or the ability to make a same-day emergency appointment), I needed to convey those needs to him, through both words and actions. I owed it to him to be honest, candid and specific, rather than guarded or vague. As much as I wanted to be agreeable and passive, he deserved to see and hear my confusion. It was useless for me to nod my head "yes" when in my head, I was thinking, "How? Why?" or "I don't understand." Just as he made allowances for my needs and concerns, I needed to consider his. He didn't deserve to have his time and energy wasted, nor did I. It took time to get comfortable with this approach to my healthcare because it felt as though I was the one making all the effort. Eventually, though, the benefits far outweighed any energy I expended.

It became second nature to prepare for my appointments, not days in advance, but for a few minutes the night before. This allowed me to clarify the questions and concerns I had in my head, rather than recalling them on the fly, erroneously or incongruently, during my visit. I got the answers I needed because now I was asking the right questions. I took notes during my appointment, demonstrating that I was indeed listening, if not analyzing, our discussion. Dr. R responded favorably to my inquisitive nature. His attentiveness increased, and his ability to connect with me and decipher my laymen's terminology improved. All around, it was as though we were both stepping up our game, each to meet the other's expectations.

I loved the ownership I felt for my own health and well-being. My actions were serving as a catalyst for better health care. It wasn't that Dr. R's care was ever substandard, but the fact that he was a smart, capable physician only went so far. I needed to feel as though he and I were in this fight together. That's exactly the way it was, now that I had become more accountable for my healing. I no longer saw Dr. R as a savior as much as I did a collaborator, an equal party who valued, wanted and needed my opinion. He was still the authority on medical issues, but I sought his advice and diagnoses with a more balanced, confident, levelheaded attitude.

Today, my appointments are livelier and less demanding, more enjoyable and less frequent. Dr. R and I spend more time talking about my interests, plans, and activities than ailments, complaints and immobility. But we still share a mutual respect and consideration for one another. Even when it comes to non-medical, unrelated issues like movies, family or travel, I know he values my opinion just as much as I do his. We communicate well, his quick wit providing a good counterpoint to my sarcastic sense of humor, even when discussing the most serious or troublesome aspects of my disease.

He has tailored my treatment as my needs and goals have shifted over time. Thus, I've never wavered from his instruction. I figure if I do my job, he can do his. He's continually tweaking and modifying aspects of my care, even when I've been healthy for months. His diligence reminds me that, in order to stay ahead of lupus, I have to stay alert. He researches and stays abreast of issues and concerns that are pertinent to my personal health and lifestyle, making me feel as though I'm the only patient he has. To this day, my daily good health is a reminder of the strong, lasting, effective relationship I've developed with my doctor. Because I've learned to hone my skills as a patient, my doctor can better address my needs as one.

Making it work

Are you ready to transform your doctor/patient relationship into a beneficial, rewarding rapport that works? Great! There are strategic ways to make the most out of each visit with your doctor, but change takes time. Every effort, no matter how small, will help lay the groundwork for a better working relationship with your physician. Before you know it, the incremental changes you've instituted will result in an improved, healthier connection with your doctor. The key is realizing just how important your actions are to the overall success of your healthcare. You owe it to yourself to make the most out of the time and energy you spend at the doctor's office, and you expect (and are desperate for) an elite performance from your doctor. You want him to be at his best when he walks into your examining room. The best way to do that is to expect the same of yourself.

Think about the times that you didn't arrive prepared for an appointment. You forgot the questions you wanted to ask, arrived late or chose not to notate the doctor's specific instructions you were to follow. Maybe you were dishonest about how closely you followed the doctor's orders or were evasive about your symptoms because you were embarrassed or ashamed. These errors in judgment might have been unintentional or seemed insignificant to you, but they have a profound effect on the way your doctor sees you as a patient. Remember, this is a partnership, and if one-half of the equation fails, so does the other half. In order to ensure the best treatment from your doctor, you need to become the best patient. Being "good" has nothing to do with the mildness of your disease or how few symptoms you present during any given visit. It's based on your willingness to collaborate, your level of engagement and your ability to be patient, prepared and responsible. Your doctor thrives on solving the medical mysteries that you bring him; let him do so by supporting, if not actively contributing, to the efforts he's making. You elevate yourself to a position of influence, one that commands respect and attention in a cooperative sort of way.

Collaborating with a physician to solve the dilemma of your disease is no different than working with a colleague to unravel the latest company crisis. In each case, successfully uniting the two key players and managing that relationship is paramount to achieving the desired result. You know how it goes: utilize the team's strengths, acknowledge the limitations, and make adjustments as needed. You and your doctor are allies, so you may have to overlook his inconsequential flaws (like his bad sense of humor or the fact that he runs 20 minutes late for his appointments) in order to take full advantage of his skills. This doesn't mean that you should excuse all of his flaws. But it does mean that, just as at work, you must learn to work around your collaborator's shortcomings.

You may need to challenge your doctor on certain issues, but making inquiries doesn't have to be confrontational. On the contrary, highlighting a difference in opinion can spark communication and ingenuity in both you and your doctor. Time spent begrudging your doctor for unresolved past conflict could be better spent focusing on the future of your health and how best to improve it. I am guilty of not resolving disputes during an appointment and then complaining about it (and my doctor) for days after. He probably didn't even know that it was a point of conflict to begin with! Most importantly, learn to put your greatest assets forward, enabling your doctor to do the same. When you're prepared, precise and truthful, it will prompt him to respond in the same manner.

My relationship with Dr. R took time and patience to develop, but it was well worth the effort. There were times when I worried about questioning his care, being too forceful, or including too much detail in explaining my symptoms. But in doing so, I let him know how eager I was to become well, and he responded by steadily (if not tirelessly) making it happen. In this chapter, you'll learn how to improve your doctor-patient relationship by using the following three guidelines to render it effective:

→ **Be Assertive**
→ **Seek Clarity**
→ **React Reasonably**

Don't just hope that you and your doctor can work well together. Expect it!

Keys to a better relationship

Let's assume for a moment that the medical care you're receiving is less than ideal. Maybe it's not a complete waste of time, but perhaps the time you spend with your doctor is absolute drudgery. You may have struggled to pinpoint what isn't working, or maybe you've identified it but don't know how to fix it. This chapter is geared toward those patients who are looking to improve the effectiveness of their doctor-patient relationship by altering their own behavior in order to maximize the results. Most issues can be prevented or even eliminated if you employ this strategy.

As with any partnership, some are salvageable; others are not. If you listen to a lupus patient complain about his/her doctor, you can usually identify within minutes whether the patient needs to modify his/her behavior (because he/she admits to self-medicating or disobeying doctor's orders, for example), or if the doctor needs to be better managed and/or ditched (due to rude, dismissive, or clashing behavior). No one should settle for substandard health care, particularly when you have the opportunity to seek out better or more suitable arrangements. The doctors who coordinate your treatment are vitally important to your health and well-being, and you should do everything in your power not to compromise that care.

1) BE ASSERTIVE

In the beginning, I hated confronting Dr. R. I wasn't afraid of him as much as I feared the answers he had to give me. I worried about articulating the questions swirling around in my head and dreaded the onslaught of tears that came so readily during those first few months. But about six months after I started seeing him, I felt that I had hit a plateau. I still was very sick and wasn't making progress. My family prompted me to seek a second opinion, but I had to tell Dr. R first so that my charts could be released. It may sound like an easy thing to do, but I was terrified. I had to tell the one person who had been my greatest advocate that after all he'd done to help me, I didn't think it was enough. I felt like a traitor and didn't think I was strong enough (mentally or physically) to go through with it.

When I finally broached the subject with him, he responded professionally and amicably, much to my relief. He agreed that it was a good idea that 'we' get a second opinion, instantly sharing the burden and making it seem as though it was a logical step. In fact, he suggested that, instead of seeking the help of the physician I'd named, we should set up an appointment at the National Institutes of Health ("NIH") with a specialist in the field. It seemed he wanted answers just as badly as I did. Had I never asserted myself, though, would he ever have suggested it?

He prepared the necessary documentation and made the appropriate phone calls and within days, I was at NIH. There, I underwent a thorough series of tests and examinations. The doctor there followed up with me several times over a period of two months, concluding that my care under Dr. R thus far had been appropriate and sufficient. Dr. R was doing everything right; lupus just wasn't responding.

I returned to Dr. R's permanent care, confident that he was doing all he could to fix me. I worried that I had offended him with my insistence to see someone else and considered the fact that our relationship might be permanently tarnished. On the contrary, it only strengthened it. Now, he saw me as a patient who meant business: someone who was straightforward and honest, self-assured and independent. I wanted to take responsibility for my health, not just accept his advice and guidance without question.

The greatest change didn't come from him; it came from me. After I witnessed his positive response to and the results of my polite, yet firm confrontation, I saw myself in a whole new light. I proved that I could be confident and definitive, even in a subject where my counterpart had the advantage. It was the first time I had taken the future of my health in my own hands, and it felt good. Having reestablished my self-confidence while earning my doctor's respect, our relationship began to thrive.

Since then, I've exhibited my assertiveness time and again with Dr. R, realizing now that he expects nothing less from me. There have been times when he seemed distracted or impatient, dismissing a symptom I'm concerned about or glossing over an issue too quickly. I try rephrasing my question or readdressing the issue in another manner, perhaps at a more appropriate time. Note that I never sacrifice my expectations; I just learn to compromise on the approach in order to get what I need. Assertiveness isn't about brawn or brute force; instead, it's about diplomatically displaying a self-confidence that cannot be ignored.

2) ASK QUESTIONS

The easiest way to assert yourself during a doctor's appointment is to verbalize your questions. In doing so, you instantly convey interest while elevating the doctor to an assumed position of authority (which he will undoubtedly appreciate.) Your query instantly sets up a framework within which both you and your doctor can begin to work. Until you speak, your doctor is left to interpret your head nods and strings of "uh-huh's" the best he can. How is he to know your nods of confirmation are actually nods of confusion? Instead of misleading your doctor, define your level of comprehension by asking a relevant question. Even if it's just repeating what your doctor has said in a question format, it will force your doctor to take pause and consider that he is indeed talking *with* you, not just at you. It also will appear that you're paying attention and engrossed, further demanding that your doctor be precise and stay sharp.

→DO YOU GET UNSPOKEN RESISTANCE WHEN YOU ASK A QUESTION?

Maybe you're not asking your questions at the most opportune time or perhaps your doctor already covered the information you're requesting. In case of the former, ask your doctor when it would be most appropriate for you to ask your questions. Suggest, for instance, the beginning, the end, or mid-appointment (when the subject is actually being discussed). He may have a preference and, if so, it's in your best interest to adhere to it. It's a simple adjustment you can make that will help you get the answers you want while not disrupting your doctor's flow.

In the case of the latter, perhaps you need to bone up on your note-taking skills. Take a pad of paper and a pen or turn to the notes section of your personal digital assistant ("PDA"). Jot down items of interest during the appointment, underlining a confusing word or phrase to remind yourself that what your doctor just said didn't make sense. When you're taking notes, your body language, or lack thereof, also may indicate what's going on in your brain. If he starts to rattle off the steps you need to take before beginning a course of medication, for example, and you don't write a thing, he'll take the cue that he needs to stop and review what he's saying. I've formed the habit of turning on my PDA, going to my notepad screen, and creating a new file or reviewing the notes that I've already made for that particular appointment before the doctor walks into the room. When he sees that my PDA is up and prepped for action, he knows I'm ready and engaged, indicating that he should be, too.

→DOES YOUR DOCTOR SPEAK TOO QUICKLY FOR YOU TO TAKE NOTES?

If so, get ready to write with your pad of paper and when your doctor's pace begins to quicken unnecessarily, immediately ask him to repeat and review. Soon enough, you'll find a pace that works for both of you. Intuitively, he may begin to slow his words when there's something that he needs to make sure you understand. If he accommodates you, make a note to thank him after the appointment. Progress and improvement shouldn't go unrecognized.

→DON'T THINK YOUR APPOINTMENTS WARRANT ANY QUESTIONS?

Maybe your doctor isn't in the room with you for more than five minutes, and you're convinced there's no time to get a word in before he's on to his next patient. I promise you that, if you show up with a pad of paper and a list of questions, you'll get some airtime. If your time is limited, make sure you prioritize and ask all of your imperative questions first. If your list is a bit long to tackle in one appointment, don't be offended if your question/answer session is cut short. Ask how it's best to get the remaining questions answered before your next appointment. Could you email him? Is there someone else in the office you could talk to today or later in the week? If the questions aren't urgent, and you have to wait until the next appointment to discuss them, that's okay. Just make it clear that during your next visit, you intend to have them answered. This can be as simple as saying, with a smile, "Okay, I'll just make sure that I pose them during my next appointment." It's not his approval you're seeking; it's an expectation you're providing. In that single sentence, you have diplomatically, yet effectively managed the situation. Be sure to follow up at the next appointment: have your pad of paper ready before the doctor comes in, reminding him that you need answers, and preferably today.

I'm sure I don't have to explain that the idea isn't to harass, inconvenience, or badger your doctor with mundane, irrelevant or inappropriate questions. In fact, it's just the opposite. You're appealing to his expertise, wisdom and knowledge – not to assert yourself for your own personal satisfaction. The objective is to improve your healthcare. If engaging in a pointed question and answer session lays the foundation for that to happen, jump at the opportunity.

You might find that your questions serve as a gentle, helpful reminder to your doctor, jogging his memory about something he needed to discuss with you. They could, in fact, prompt an entire conversation that might not have otherwise taken place. This happened to me recently, when my mother-in-law, out of curiosity, asked how my doctor planned on reducing a certain medication I was planning to discontinue that summer. Would it happen all at once or would I taper off over the course of a few months? In all of the discussions Dr. R. and I had about that particular prescription change, we'd never spoken of this minor detail. I made a note to ask him at my next appointment. Sure enough, when I posed the question to him, he had an entire strategy planned out for how I was to taper off the medication. He and I immediately decided to start tapering off sooner than he'd originally planned in order to reach our target end date. I'm sure the issue eventually would have come up, but thank goodness for inquisitive in-laws to move the process along!

3) TAKE SOMEONE ALONG

When you're really sick, maintaining an animated discussion, full of provoking questions, can seem impossible. You may feel as though you're lessening the effectiveness of your appointments. If so, consider taking someone in with you. It's important that you choose your companion carefully, as you don't want to feel inhibited by his/her presence. Nor do you want your companion to be unnerved by the detailed discussions that might occur. Once you have the right person by your side, you'll be reassured to know that someone else is there to listen, interpret and, if you choose, speak on your behalf. From time to time, I've asked my husband or sister to accompany me to my appointments. When that happens, Dr. R knows that something is amiss. He's even joked that when I walk in the door with a companion, he knows he's "in trouble." Granted, I tend to bring in my back-up troops when I feel I'm not getting through to him or when I've been sick for weeks without explanation. Yet, the presence of a third party seems to be just the stimulus we both need to renew a direct and effective line of communication.

I had the opportunity once to accompany my girlfriend, Carol, to Dr. R's office, and it was a truly eye-opening experience. For one thing, I jotted down more notes than I ever had during one of my appointments. I was conscious of the fact that she had asked me to be there for support as well as a second set of ears. In addition, I was able to see Dr. R from the perspective of a layperson, not as a patient with a long list of needs and concerns. Because Carol had never seen Dr. R before, the majority of her appointment was spent in his actual office, simply talking about her health history.

For thirty minutes, she revealed the trials, tribulations, and symptoms she'd experienced with lupus, including the courses of medications, tests and procedures she'd undergone. Dr. R asked a few questions, but he primarily scribbled down indecipherable, random notes on a single sheet of unlined paper throughout the discussion. Once a new patient myself, I remember sitting in that office with Johnny by my side, divulging my entire life's story to, then, a perfect stranger. I was unsure of what information the doctor wanted or needed, and I struggled to articulate or recall the chronology of all of the crazy symptoms I had experienced. I remember trying hard not to censor my story due to ignorance or unfamiliarity, though I was suffering from both. I remembered being impressed with what Dr. R did after I finished my chronicles but, at the time, I was too sick and overwhelmed to appreciate his aptitude. Here, I had a chance to see it again from an entirely different perspective.

After Carol was done, Dr. R turned on his handy recording device into which he records a summation of every appointment. He began to recount with precision, a concise, medically accurate narration of Carol's journey with lupus while, on the fly, interjecting his own medical inferences, suppositions, and deductions. Given my familiarity with the disease, I experienced many of the things about which she had spoken. To me, they were just as inexplicable, unfortunate and random as she thought they were. But he had miraculously assembled those complex, disjointed facts into a compact, sensible, orderly story, giving her lifelong pain and suffer-ing definition, identity and meaning. It was an extraordinary feat and, all at once, I had the opportunity to see, in part, how and why he had been so effective during the three years that I'd been seeing him. I even may have benefited from that ap-pointment more than my friend did!

I had another chance to sit in on a doctor's appointment that wasn't my own, this time accompanying my sister to a doctor's visit about which she was particularly nervous. We discussed some of the questions she planned to ask on the way to the appointment. Like a good, prepared patient, she'd brought a list of things she wanted to mention to the doctor. Several minutes into the appointment, though, I could tell that her brain was becoming overloaded with all of the information discussed, just as mine would and usually does during my own appointments. As she'd done for me dozens of times in the past, I jumped in and asked a few ques-tions myself, relieving her of the pressure and/or confusion one feels when the issue of your own health is being discussed. On our drive home, I helped her re-cap the discussion that had taken place, remembering a few details that she had forgotten. I realized how beneficial she'd been during my sickest visits to my doc-tor, and I was happy to repay the favor.

Here is one last example of how beneficial it can be to have a second set of ears during a doctor's visit. During a recent check-up, a friend of mine complained to his doctor of digestive trouble. The doctor recommended he make a certain addition to his diet, to which he adhered for the next six weeks. He went back for a follow-up appointment, this time accompanied by his wife. Having stayed apprised of her husband's dietary changes, she immediately asked the doctor how much longer her husband needed to eat the eight plums a day he had prescribed. "Eight plums?" the doctor exclaimed. "I said *a* plum!" Who knows if she would have correctly heard the doctor at the previous appointment, but my bet is her presence would have helped!

4) SEEK CLARITY THROUGH RECAP AND REVIEW

As I alluded to earlier, my doctor uses a funny little recording device at the end of each appointment to document everything that's been discussed. While I now understand how sensible, even vital, it is to rehash the finer points of an appointment, I'd never seen a professional use a tape recorder before. In the beginning, it just seemed so melodramatic and over-the-top. Whenever he would launch into his full-bore recap of an appointment, I would avoid making eye contact and do my best to suppress my laughter. Who knows why it was so funny back then, watching him speak into a little recorder about all of the terrible things that were happening to my body. Maybe it was the novelty, but I imagine the routine allowed me just a few minutes to refocus my thoughts, not toward myself, but on him. Here was an intelligent, experienced, highly respected physician in whom I had put my complete faith, hope and trust, and he was struggling to speak normally into this teeny, tiny little recorder. He'd start speaking, then stop, rewind, rephrase his words, and start over again. He'd repeat and stumble over words, often tripping over the easiest phrases. I would have the same trouble, of course; the task of recording's one voice always seems daunting.

At the end of each recording session, Dr. R enumerates my action items between appointments. Whether I need to start (or stop) a prescription, get an X-ray, see another doctor, or watch for symptoms to change or arise, it's all recapped at this time. It's the perfect way to summarize what has happened, what needs to happen and, in some cases, what should happen. The conclusion of the recording session is the definitive moment when we can look each other in the eye and confirm that, yes, with absolute certainty, doctor and patient agree. In fact, it's like a temporary reversal of roles, where I get to be the teacher and he, the student. He gives the oral report and then I grade him on it. It is Dr. R's moment in the spotlight, the few minutes during which he tries to recount everything we've discussed while I sit back, "testing" his recall. In most cases, he records the details accurately. In the rare event that he misses something, I signal for him to stop, I correct his mistake (or ask for clarification), and then he continues. I used to only half-listen as he repeated the happenings of our appointment, but I soon realized that this simple, albeit amusing, exercise is as much for my benefit as it is for his.

I overheard a phone conversation between him and an evidently frustrated, confused patient once. She was denying that he'd prescribed a medication to her and he said according to the dictation, he had. Didn't she remember him mentioning it at that time? He expects his patients to listen intently, correcting his mistakes and double-checking his work, and I'm happy to oblige.

Even if your doctor doesn't utilize a tape recorder, it's still possible to get a summary at the end of every visit. Simply ask your doctor to review the highlights or repeat the action items to which you (or he) have been assigned. If you prefer, you can even recount the details to him. That will ensure that you have your facts straight.

Don't be too hard on yourself if you find that you've missed significant parts of the appointment. I never realized how disoriented I was during my sickest appointments until recently. I made an appointment to see someone other than my primary doctor in my perinatologist's office, thinking I was seeing someone new. At the start of the appointment with her, I immediately launched into my entire medical history as it related to lupus and pregnancy. Halfway through my story, she pointed out that I didn't need to rehash my history. She actually had seen me before. In fact, she'd performed an outpatient surgery and had followed up with me several times afterward. Those previous appointments had taken place during the early stages of a bad flare and in the midst of a miscarriage, so I definitely wasn't as alert as I could have been. Thankfully, she understood my haziness and wasn't offended!

It's understandable if you're not as coherent as you'd like to be during your appointments. Just be honest with yourself, and realize you may need to prepare or take extra steps to ensure that you're getting the most out of your visit with the doctor. You should benefit from every appointment, both parties working in unison to ensure a successful outcome and a healthier, happier you!

5) BE HONEST AND SPECIFIC

Because lupus is not a disease that is easily treated, your doctor needs all the help he can get in order to make an accurate diagnosis. Your visits to the doctor may include a good deal of trial and error as it is, and you don't want to complicate the matter by being vague or deceitful about the symptoms you experience. An honest and upfront approach is the only way your doctor can obtain the information he needs to make a diagnosis of your unpredictable, evasive disease. He has no choice but to analyze only those symptoms he detects at the time of your appointment or those of which you inform him. If you fail to mention the hip pain you had yesterday, the swelling in your fingers over the weekend, or the hair loss you've noticed in the shower, he's not going to have a complete picture of how the disease is currently manifesting. No matter how embarrassed or inhibited you may feel, it's imperative that you put those emotions aside. You need to equip your doctor with the facts in order to get results.

I remember a specific example when I had an ill placed, embarrassing rash on, you guessed it, my buttocks. I was reluctant to tell my doctor about it because I was self-conscious about showing him where it was and what it looked like. I was also a little afraid of hearing why it was there in the first place. I finally mustered up the courage to mention it to him, and upon seeing it, he concluded that it might be attributed to an infection in my bloodstream. I was put on both an oral and topical medication to eradicate the rash, and I quickly learned that, in the future, I might have to put pride aside in order to enable my doctor to do his job effectively.

Maybe you're self-conscious about the fact that you've been self-medicating or straying from doctors orders, neither of which are productive practices. They become even more damaging, however, when you deny that you're doing them. How is your doctor going to accurately gauge your progress (or regression) from one appointment to another if he's under the illusion that you're taking medication or abstaining from activities that you're really not? It's paramount that you be honest and upfront, not only with your doctor, but with yourself as well.

I shared a hospital room with a woman who, for three days, lied to her doctors about the fact that she was smoking. She announced to me at least twice a day that she was leaving the room to go have a cigarette and, every day, I would overhear the convincing claims she fed her doctor, confirming that, no, she hadn't had a cigarette since the day she was admitted. She was working against the very people who were working so hard to help her. While I don't condone her actions, I know how easy it is to convince yourself that you're in compliance with doctor's orders, even when you're not. For months, I would adamantly profess to Dr. R that I was doing everything I could to get better – following his instructions, taking my medication, staying out of the sun. What I didn't mention were the 50 hour work weeks I was putting in, my reluctance to slow down when I felt feverish, and the vacations I continued to take even though I felt weak and sickly. He never asked those questions directly, so I never told him. Ambiguity had morphed into what is more aptly called dishonesty. It was hurting everyone involved. Allow yourself to capitalize on the expertise of your doctor by offering up all of the information you can.

6) REACT REASONABLY

Take a moment to consider how many physicians you've seen since you were diagnosed with lupus. They each have their own style, don't they? I've seen more than a dozen specialists since lupus came into my life, each of whom have poked, prodded and prescribed a little differently than the last. No two doctors are alike, and yet our hope (and maybe even expectation) is the same each time we visit: cure me now. We turn to our medical team with eagerness and expectancy because we believe they can and will provide the solutions we need. It's comforting to put such faith in the profession as a whole, but it's important that we remember the individuality of each doctor. Consider how their distinctiveness might mesh with your own uniqueness as a patient. You have a subconscious expectation that the two will work in harmony. When they don't, it can be off-putting and a little disheartening.

Instead of becoming discouraged, acknowledge that your relationship may need a little finessing in order to be successful. Managing people takes a great deal of patience, understanding and skill, and that's how you should approach the relationship with your medical professionals. You should think of it not in a controlling, autocratic manner, but with a level of tolerance and perceptiveness that will allow you to juggle personalities, behaviors and agendas with proven effectiveness. Perhaps you're concerned that by accepting another person's personality quirks, you'll be lowering your expectations for effective health care. That's not the case at all. Acknowledging that people's temperaments and personalities don't always match allows you to stop blaming yourself (or your health care provider) for the futility you experience from your appointments. Having established that no one in particular is at fault, you can objectively evaluate your care in order to improve it.

Doctors are real people, too

Just like you and me, your doctor is only human. He has strengths and weaknesses, assets and imperfections. He's going to have good days and bad days and because you see him as frequently as you do, you're bound to catch him on one of each. Your doctor should always conduct himself professionally (even on his worst day). But it's unrealistic to expect him to overhaul his behavior simply to meet your personal expectations. You may want more small talk and less business; a shoulder to cry on instead of a composed, unemotional handshake; or more supportive encouragement and less brutal honesty. Just because that's what you want doesn't mean your doctor is responsible for giving it to you. In fact, he may be incapable of relating to you in that way. If that is the case, you may need to learn to accept your doctor for his expertise *and* his failings - or switch doctors.

A friend of mine, Marjorie, was in the middle of an appointment when she discovered a weakness that her beloved, accomplished, competent doctor had. During the course of this particular appointment, her doctor delivered some very bad news. Marjorie instantly broke down in tears, crying hysterically. Her doctor was visually uncomfortable during the outburst and was speechless. She didn't reach out to console or comfort Marjorie, and it was as if she was incapable of behaving normally in the presence of a sobbing, panicked patient. It was a side of her doctor that Marjorie had never seen before, and she was shocked. Once Marjorie calmed down and composed herself, the doctor resumed her formidable personality, communicating intelligently and astutely, with no sign of the stunted, inhibited traits she had just exhibited moments earlier. Marjorie concluded that, while she certainly could have used some words of consolation during her outburst, her doctor was far too valuable to let this small, relatively workable issue get in the way of a successful relationship.

I, too, have learned to adjust to Dr. R's occasional tendency to be insensitive. I experience (and appreciate) his kind and caring traits much more often than his terse disposition. However, some days, his crisp, undemonstrative nature is just the thing I need to keep my emotions in check. I remember a particular instance when, just six short months after I'd gotten married, Dr. R needed to make it clear that I had to avoid becoming pregnant for the benefit of my own personal well-being. As a newlywed, it was one of the most devastating things I'd ever been told. Of course, I wasn't actively trying to get pregnant, nor was I planning to start anytime soon. Yet, the fact that lupus was restricting me at all caused me to start tearing up. Thankfully, Dr. R didn't turn the situation into a big emotional production. He gently explained what the dangers were if I did become pregnant, letting me collect myself as he kept me focused on the facts. While his face and tone of voice conveyed his consolation, his reserved nature kept my tears at bay. He succeeded in preventing an unnecessary breakdown.

IS IT WORKING?
Decide for yourself

Are you still troubled by a rocky doctor-patient connection? All relationships require some amount of effort, but the payoff should undoubtedly equal the energy you're putting forth. If you spend an inordinate amount of time trying to make peace with your doctor, or if the differences between the two of you are interfering with the effectiveness of your medical treatment, it may be time to switch physicians. It doesn't matter how many shining referrals, write-ups, or reviews your doctor has to his name. You should never settle for substandard, dissatisfying or unsettling care. The most important evaluation is the one you give him, and if you're not happy with the results, you're entitled to try someone else.

Use these questions to help you pinpoint what is not working in your current relationship:

- **What are your greatest needs from a physician?**
- **What are your expectations?**
- **Have you brought them to his attention?**
- **Is your current doctor capable or incapable of meeting those needs and expectations?**
- **Could you help him do so in a more effective way than you currently are?**
- **What are your personality strengths and weaknesses?**
- **How might they complement or clash with those of your physician?**

Let's not forget about the more tangible considerations that might inhibit or enhance a visit to the doctor. While it may not be prudent to base the value of your medical care on generic issues, like whether or not a doctor takes after-hours calls, it is important to establish your expectations and consider your preferences. You may find one factor to be irrelevant to you, while another factor weighs heavily on how pleasant or unpleasant a visit to the doctor may become.

Consider the following, keeping in mind that every aspect of your appointment, from the commute to the co-pay, makes a difference in how you view your overall satisfaction with your doctor:

- Ease and comprehensiveness of insurance coverage
- Proximity of the office to your home/work
- Ability to schedule an appointment on short notice
- Approximate wait time per visit
- Number of doctors in the practice
- Office hours
- Doctor accessibility (email, pager, after hours contact)
- Affiliated hospitals
- Laboratory work done in-house
- Reputation
- Parking, elevators, handicap accessibility, etc.

In the case that you do decide to try another doctor, be sure that you've been honest with yourself about what wasn't working in the original relationship. By pinpointing your concerns, you make it easier to discern whether the next doctor is better suited to meet your needs. You also might consider the appropriateness of discussing why you're leaving with your current doctor. If it's a personality clash or a matter of personal preference, there's probably no need to burden your doctor with the concern. If it's a more serious matter that needs to be brought to his (or someone else's) attention (*e.g.* unacceptable or illegal behavior), do so as diplomatically as possible.

Other helpful hints

→ **CREATE YOUR OWN MEDICAL NETWORK:** Make an effort to keep all doctors informed of your other appointments, tests, and treatments. Begin by requesting that test results and appointment minutes be shared amongst the doctors managing your care. At the very least, make a note to yourself to mention the results or information during your next appointment. Enable your doctors to begin working together by informing each of them who your other doctors are. It may not be necessary for them to converse often. However, keeping them apprised of your network of health providers, as well as the status of your health, will give you the reassurance of knowing that your doctors are managing your health care collectively and cooperatively. This will ideally provide you with a check and balance system that will ease your burden and optimize your care.

→ **UTILIZE YOUR NETWORK:** Never hesitate to consult a medical professional about a problem you're experiencing, even if it's a known side effect of your disease. For example, hair loss and food allergies are both known side effects of lupus. For all too long, I convinced myself that I just had to live with these issues. Now I know that I should have consulted a dermatologist or seen an allergist at the start of my trouble. Even if the solutions available to me were limited, I would have saved myself the torment and frustration of toughing it out or diagnosing myself. Be it acne, weight gain, scarring or some other problem caused by your medication or the disease itself, don't hesitate to call upon the resources available to you. Get the help you deserve and save yourself further trouble.

→ **CHOOSE A NETWORK CAPTAIN:** When possible, choose a doctor who can help you coordinate and keep tabs on your lupus treatment as a whole. This doesn't need to be a formal arrangement, nor does your doctor need to do anything more than what he would normally do. This is primarily for your benefit, so that you have a main point of contact for all things related to lupus. Choose a doctor with whom you have a good relationship and one who is well suited for the job (*i.e.* intimately involved with your lupus care). This can be any doctor you choose, mine happens to be my rheumatologist, my girlfriend's is her gynecologist, and another's is her primary care physician. Once you've designated your "captain," use that doctor to help you keep all other doctors well informed of your disease activity. Let that doctor be your confidant and sounding board, not for complaints or unnecessary rants, but as a person to whom you can turn with questions, concerns, or confusion when it comes to lupus. They may refer you to another doctor, but at least they can get you on the right track. You'll soon begin to see what a relief is to have an expert leading the way and on your side.

Good doctors are out there

Upon diagnosis, you may have thought that finding and working with a good doctor would be the least of your chronic illness concerns. After all, good doctors are everywhere, and lupus isn't the newest disease on the block. Truth is, we want it to be an easy process, but it can actually be one of the hardest aspects of dealing with your disease. It can require a great amount of energy to locate, schedule and establish treatment with a good and reputable doctor. Even then, you aren't guaranteed a relationship that works.

You should not think of the relationship with your primary chronic illness doctor as fleeting. You're not looking to have a few good appointments and then move on; you have to count on a lifetime of follow-up, sprinkled (or laden) with difficulty and complication. You can't face all that with just anyone! Developing an effective doctor-patient connection takes time and energy, but the benefit of making such a significant effort will prove itself almost immediately.

One of my doctors confessed that he thought every doctor would benefit from having a chronic illness. He said they would then experience for themselves the mental and physical distress and agony that patients with diseases like lupus undergo. He was sincere in his comments and, while I don't wish lupus on anyone, he has a point. We can't expect our doctors to comprehend what it's like to live with a chronic illness. That's why it's our job to work closely with them so that they can assess, diagnose and solve our problems as efficiently as possible. Assisting your doctor in this way doesn't have to take much, but it can save you loads of time, money and frustration.

I have benefited greatly from my efforts to understand Dr. R. Today, my relationship with him is effortless. You, of all people, need an effective doctor-patient relationship that works. I know you have the common sense, perseverance and patience to make it happen. Good doctors are out there, you just have to know how to find them, work with them and, most importantly, make them work for you.

CHAPTER 5: COMMUNICATE WISELY

I attended my first lupus support group meeting nearly six months after my diagnosis. I'd learned early on that there was a group in my area and even had the contact information of the group's facilitator. But I had no intention of ever attending a meeting, so I shoved the scrap paper with her phone number on it into the back of a book where I could forget about it. I wasn't interested in sitting around a table filled with desperate, depressed, sickly people, most of whom were surely far worse off than I was. I'm sure they were fine people, but I'd read enough about the potential consequences of having lupus; I didn't need to *see* them in full effect. I also didn't want other people's negativity to rub off on me. I was fighting to stay positive on my own and saw no benefit in listening to a bunch of strangers try and convince me to feel sorry for myself or for them. In fact, I wasn't even ready to admit that I was officially sick, much less discuss the fact in a group-like setting.

It wasn't that I didn't believe in seeking help in a support group. My dad had been participating in semi-weekly, 12-step group meetings for over twenty years, and the benefits for him of doing so had been obvious. From time to time, my mom, sister and I attended our own affiliated group meetings. There, I personally experienced the empowerment that comes from surrounding yourself with supportive, understanding, like-minded individuals.

Based upon this positive experience, you'd think I would have been eager to join a group that could have provided that same kind of support. To the contrary, the idea of attending a meeting left me feeling anxious and uneasy. It wasn't just the condition of the people in the group that I was worried about. I knew that if I went, I would be admitting that I was too weak to deal with lupus on my own. I would no longer appear resilient or self-sufficient, not to others, or to myself. That sense of independence was vital to me, and I wasn't going to do anything to endanger that freedom.

However, my family strongly encouraged me to find out more about the meetings. I decided that contacting the facilitator would appease them, but wouldn't commit me to anything, so I gathered up the courage to make the call to Gail, the coordinator. I learned that the next meeting was a mere two weeks away and would take place at a library not more than twenty minutes from my house – it couldn't have been more convenient. Yet when I got off the phone, I immediately conjured up a dozen excuses why I shouldn't go. Could I really afford the time to attend? Hadn't I been feeling a little better lately? What would I even have to contribute? I wasn't willing to talk about the complaints and concerns I had, and certainly not to a bunch of strangers. I had perfected the art of keeping all apprehension and uncertainty to myself. I thought my anger, resentment, and vulnerability needed to stay buried, as they would only slow me down or create a burden for someone else.

I doubted if anyone around me would understand my predicament anyway. No one could even grasp that the more they doted on me, the more threatened and inadequate I felt. Lupus was stripping me of my pride and dignity, and their sympathy only made me feel worse. I didn't want to complicate the situation by voluntarily joining a group whose purpose was to commiserate with one another.

When the day of the meeting arrived, I realized that this actually might be an opportunity to demonstrate just how out of place I would be in a group like this. I asked my husband and sister to accompany me and looked forward to proving my point. But when we arrived at the library, I was much less confident than I thought I'd be. I felt my heart quicken and my chest tighten as we walked toward the meeting room. Upon entering, I glanced around the table and was puzzled. From the looks of those gathered together, I knew this couldn't be a lupus meeting. There wasn't a sick face in the group. I was proven wrong as a sharply dressed woman came forward and introduced herself as Gail, the coordinator I'd spoken to. She invited us to sit down, and then asked everyone to introduce themselves.

As each person described how they were diagnosed with lupus, I noted the absence of even one sob story. These women weren't lamenting the fact they had the disease, they were dealing with it with dignity, just the way I envisioned myself doing. The stories they told sounded like my story: a diagnosis out of the blue, total shock to their lifestyle, a struggle to make the symptoms work with their life's plan. Listening to them talk about the same symptoms and emotions with which I'd grown so familiar gave me an overwhelming sense of comfort and security. In fact, everything they said made me feel validated. Here was a group of ordinary, well-adjusted people, trying to deal with the inconvenience of lupus, just like I was. It was like walking into a world where everyone spoke the same language.

It had been a long time since I'd felt understood. Since being diagnosed, I had found it difficult to explain what it was like to have lupus to those who didn't. The physical difficulties were hard enough to describe, but the mental hurdles I encountered were incommunicable. No one close to me could grasp why my ego had been bruised or why I was struggling so hard to prove myself. They also couldn't understand why their concerns were suffocating me. And, yet, as the stories unfolded that evening during the meeting, I heard one person after another expound on the difficulty of accepting the limitations of lupus and the challenge of communicating that struggle to friends and family. These people knew exactly what it felt like to have a successful life threatened by an unannounced and unwelcome disease.

My husband and sister continued to attend the next few meetings with me out of consideration, but soon enough, I encouraged them to stop joining me. I relished the personal time I had with the group each month. It was a time when I could work through my biggest lupus stumbling blocks in the companionship and camaraderie of those who could relate. We talked about the trivial parts of our everyday life with the same fervor as the serious, significant aspects of lupus. Traveling the world, competing in marathons and finding the best new restaurants in town were just as important as discussing the latest drugs or procedures in the chronic-illness market. The candid banter was refreshing; I was tired of hyper-focusing on lupus. When people ask so persistently how you're feeling or how the disease is progressing, one starts to wonder if the disease is suddenly the only thing people see when they look at you. Thankfully, the topics discussed during our meetings ran far deeper than that, making me feel part of a well-rounded, varied, active community of people. We were normal, accomplished people first, and lupus patients second.

As my confidence grew month after month, I became less defensive and guarded about my feelings and emotions, both in and out of the meetings. In support group discussions, I found myself reaching out to others, endorsing their stories and even sharing my own. If I thought my past experiences might help someone muddle through theirs, I eagerly offered up the details of my trials with lupus. Things like refusing help from friends because of pride or pushing too hard to prove myself were common topics of discussion. I encouraged them to make better choices and decided I should do the same.

I began to make the same transformation in my personal life that I encouraged others to make in the group. I learned to capitalize on the support and encouragement others offered instead of deliberately shutting them out. I had to force myself to embrace their sympathy, but it was worth it. While I thought lupus was something I needed to conquer on my own, those around me wanted nothing more than to help me overcome it. They wanted to relieve my pain, improve my quality of life and alleviate my worries. It wasn't until I heard the stories of caretakers trying to do the same that I saw what a disservice I was doing my own family.

My self-image had been too wrapped up in what I was capable of accomplishing on my own, and I knew it. I worked to dispel my own hang-ups about feeling compromised or pathetic when someone else did something for me. With my new outlook, my relationships improved and so did my health. As others willingly took on errands too taxing for me, I had (and made) more time to rest and relax. In short, I began taking care of myself.

Embracing others in my healing process was not an easy adjustment to make. Not everyone was as empathetic as the people in my lupus group. Of course, the members of my group didn't know me before I had lupus. Their impression of me was based on the determined, young soldier they saw desperately trying to survive lupus. They had nothing to compare it to. But my friends and family had a comparison to make, and their altered view of who I was becoming left them befuddled. I could see them struggling to figure out how they fit into this new scenario. The assumption that I was an entirely different person offended me, but it was important that I consider two things: why did their opinions make me so mad and why did they think as they did? These weren't insignificant issues to confront, but uncovering the reasons gave me the perspective I needed to start making adjustments to the way I related to others. I was better equipped to show them how, when and where they could help me, free of injury or insult.

The benefits of involving others in your healing process are immeasurable, but doing so can be overwhelming. In this chapter, we'll explore:

→ **The advantages, as well as the challenges, involved with that emotional embrace**

→ **The common misconceptions that occur between you and your loved ones**

→ **The solutions for alleviating the friction that has developed**

Relationship building requires patience and skill. Be prepared to put both to work!

The benefits of engaging others through open communication

It's difficult for me to imagine my struggle with lupus without the supportive, encouraging, caring people I had around me. I was completely enveloped by friends and family willing to do anything in their power to make me well. Their compassion and attentiveness played a major role in my recovery. I know my healing process wouldn't have come as easily or as quickly without that outpouring.

The support I received was truly amazing. My husband and sister physically and mentally helped me get through each and every day. My parents and in-laws stayed in constant contact, assuring me that Johnny and I could count on them for anything. My co-workers were accommodating and understanding, making it easy for me to float in and out of work as needed. Friends cleaned my house, cooked us meals, and ran errands. They sent cards, care packages, and inspirational books. My priest sent vials of holy water from around the world, as did a perfect stranger who had heard from my Dad that I was in need of extra prayers. Family, friends and more strangers collectively donated over $24,000 to the Arthritis Foundation in honor of a marathon my family and I walked in Dublin, Ireland. Included in almost every donation was a letter filled with hope and encouragement. I am blessed to have received such kindness and know it helped restore me to the healthful life I have today.

Perhaps you're just as lucky to have a supportive network around you, or maybe those close to you are willing to give, but you're finding it difficult to receive. I sheepishly admit that, from time to time, the attention I received was overwhelming, and I didn't always know how to accept the goodwill. I wasn't used to depending on other people, and the feeling that I was incapable of taking care of myself wasn't a comfortable one.

From time to time, you may need to remind yourself just how beneficial and empowering it can be to engage others in your struggle with lupus. Here are just a few reasons why embracing the help of others is a good idea:

1) INCREASED SUPPORT

The better you are at communicating your needs to others, the more likely you are to get the help you need. And whether it's physical assistance or mental encouragement, which of us doesn't benefit from a helping hand now and again? You have lupus, which tends to leave you feeling depleted, isolated and rundown. Let yourself experience the boost of energy and the restoration of hope that comes from letting someone else help you. You'll find strength in knowing that others care and be reminded of the fact that you're not alone in your fight with lupus. There are people knocking down your door to help you; your job is to let them in.

Physical support

EXAMPLES:
Someone opening a door, running your errands, or relieving you of a chore.

Perhaps it's against your nature to accept help doing things, such as bagging your groceries at the supermarket. Realize that sharing your burden is not a reflection of your ability (or inability) as a human being. In fact, accepting help is a sign that you're a mature adult capable of knowing your body's limitations. Instead of berating yourself for "shirking" your responsibilities, rejoice in the fact that you are smart enough to prioritize and fortunate enough to be able to delegate those duties as necessary. Allowing someone to clean your home may give you the extra time (and energy) needed to share story time with your kids. Doling out tasks at work might let you contribute at the office in other ways that were never possible with your heavier workload. Lightening your physical burdens will actually give you the rest and relaxation you need in order to recoup lost moments in other parts of your life. In fact, this is such an important step along the path to living well that the next chapter is devoted entirely to asking for and accepting physical assistance.

Emotional support

Examples:

A friend sending a card, coming by to chat, or sharing an empathetic, personal experience.

The emotional support you receive from those who call, send notes, or visit is invaluable. Reading a single email from a friend who just wanted to let you know she was thinking of you may be enough to get you through the rest of that day. Don't think you have to face life's most overwhelming obstacles alone. Instead, accept the comfort and consolation that others have to offer, knowing that it's making you a stronger, more capable warrior every step of the way.

2) VALUE OF ANOTHER VIEWPOINT

When you have as intense and intimate a relationship with a disease as you do, it's difficult to make unbiased, unemotional decisions. You're embroiled in the fight of your life, therefore compromising your impartiality. You're too accustomed to the pain, the pills and the discomfort to know when "enough is enough."

It may be impossible for you to overcome your bias completely; after all, it is your body. Realize that at this point, you're incapable of having an honest, objective point of view and acknowledge the missing link that those around you might provide. Considering another person's perspective doesn't obligate you to accept or adopt all aspects of his/her stance. Instead, entertaining that person's viewpoint can enlighten, inform and encourage. At the very least, you'll be equipped to form a better, more balanced perspective of your health.

Years ago, my sister and I went home to Indiana to help my mom recover from emergency triple by-pass heart surgery. I was sicker than I'd ever been, suffering from fainting spells, nausea and high fevers, in addition to the typical pain and fatigue. Nevertheless, I was determined to be there for my mom in her time of need, so I made the flight home without hesitating. My sister had hounded me to do something about the decline in my health before we left, but I felt like she was interfering. Yes, I was sick, but it was time to focus on my mom's health right now, not my own.

Once we arrived at the hospital where my mom was, I was unable to contribute because of my condition. Instead, I kept my mom company in the bed next to hers while my dad, sister and hospital staff nursed the two of us back to health. My mom, despite her own difficulties, took notice of my ill health, citing how atypical my symptoms seemed to be during this particular flare. She wasn't overly insistent or forceful about her opinions (she couldn't be in her condition), but rather couched her comments in such a way that didn't make me defensive. Her agreeable approach let me contemplate what she was saying and deep down, I knew she was right. Her calm, seemingly unprejudiced comments allowed me to see the situation a little more clearly. For the first time, I was able to acknowledge that the confluence of symptoms I had had all summer: dizziness, unrelenting fatigue, fever, stomach pain, loss of appetite, inability to walk more than a few steps at a time and internal bleeding that presented itself each time I went to the restroom were not normal. The fact that I had arrived at the airport and immediately needed a wheelchair had left me unfazed, but my mom's objective opinion of saying, "Something isn't right," somehow hit home.

Later that day, my mom joined forces with my dad and sister, all of whom persuaded me to seek help immediately upon my return home. Unbeknownst to me, they had already called Dr. R to see whether or not they should admit me into a hospital in Indiana or if I should fly home and see him the following day. His recommendation was to fly me home on a non-stop flight and to follow up with him immediately the next day. Upon evaluating my condition, he immediately admitted me into the hospital for further testing. Within hours of admission, I had a blood transfusion, started intravenous steroids and was put on a clear liquid diet. I was there for a full week, diagnosed with lupus-induced pancreatitis and severe anemia. Throughout my week's stay, I had countless x-rays and an endoscopy and I was introduced to and monitored closely by several doctors. Upon discharge, I was down to 100 pounds, my body just skin and bones after the trauma it had experienced. When my doctor released me, he explained how very sick I'd become and how close of a call this was. Unfortunately, I had become too accustomed to my symptoms to see how severely ill I'd been.

To contemplate what might have happened if my mom hadn't been so attuned to the decline in my health is an unproductive exercise, but I'm very thankful she was. Her diplomatic intervention reminded me just how advantageous (and painless) it can be to consider someone else's viewpoint. It was just unfortunate that, up until then, I had been opposed to listening to those same recommendations my sister and husband were making.

I admit that opinions and advice don't always come in the same considerate and constructive packaging that my mom used. I bet under normal conditions, she might have been a little more forceful than she was. Thankfully, for both of us, her period of recovery made us both more approachable. Later in the chapter, we'll discuss why it seems people aren't always so tactful and what you can do to help them use more finesse.

3) RECIPROCATION

Letting someone help you enables you to, in turn, help someone else. When I first started attending my lupus group meetings, I did so because I needed advice and guidance from people who knew what I was going through. Over time, their wisdom and insight enabled me to become a healthier, happier, more balanced individual. Today, I want to share that experience with others so they, too, can benefit from the assistance I received years ago. I go to my meetings today, not desperate for help, but ready to help others in their time of need. The learning process hasn't ended; it's just been enhanced by the ability to share and discuss my own experiences with others, in an effort to improve life with lupus.

Perhaps your self-esteem has been bankrupt and your sense of purpose lost. You may think that giving in to someone else's help will only make you feel worse, more helpless and less dignified. Try looking at it from an entirely different angle. By allowing someone to give you the necessary boost to make it through the day, you're equipping yourself to help someone else down the road. Good deeds are contagious. Why not let the string of goodwill begin with you? By opening yourself up to the assistance of another, you may be jumpstarting a positive chain of events that leaves you more fulfilled and rewarded than ever before.

The challenges of engaging others through open communication

As awkward as you may find it to engage others in your healing process, those around you may be just as out of practice at being embraced! It may be difficult for them to figure out how best to demonstrate their care and concern toward you. In fact, their inherent compassion may not be conveyed in the way they intend or in the fashion that you would prefer. Thus, it's important to consider the reasons why this adjustment period is difficult.

1) YOUR OPTIMISM MAY BE MISINTERPRETED

To begin with, you may feel that your friends and family don't willingly share your optimistic attitude. You interpret their hesitancy to back your "full steam ahead" attitude as skepticism. Don't they think you can kick this thing? Are they doubtful of your ability, your strength and your willingness to fight for what you want? You detect their concerned reluctance and immediately get defensive. Why can't they see that you're attempting to rise above, rather than wallow in the pain? You refuse to be like so many others stricken with illness: the complainers and the hypochondriacs. You will not become one of *those* people, but your loved ones' apprehensions are making it more difficult for you to do so. They keep haranguing you to slow down, call the doctor, or let the laundry go. What they don't understand is that their suggestions sound more like criticism than encouragement. Their admonishments take on a condescending tone, making you fully aware of the lack of trust they have in you. Every time they say, "Don't overdo," it feels like a slap in the face, a direct attack on your ability to manage your own life and health. Instead of empowering you to make a good, healthful decision, their implications squash any sense of empowerment or support you might have hoped to glean from them.

> **❝❝** *To assume that people have within themselves the capacity to decide what is best for them is a vote of confidence.* [1]

Thus, you need to teach them to express their concern without infuriating you even more. You must show them how it feels when they attempt to "help" because they may not know the damage they are causing. Explain the negative effect their words have on you and suggest ways they can express their concern that are more encouraging to you. Remember, their advice to take it easy is justified; you're simply asking them to finesse the delivery of their message so that you're not too offended to listen.

2) YOU MAY BE MORE SENSITIVE

The magnitude of what you're grappling with goes far beyond what those around you can see on the surface. The mental and emotional strings attached to what you do (or don't do) are invisible. Even the most benign suggestion, like urging you to slow down, can feel threatening. Where they see easy adjustments, you see your life being ripped apart. Not only do you feel that your abilities are being tested, but so are your feelings of adequacy and worthiness. What good are you if you can't accomplish the things you think you should? Being asked not to work so hard or do so much is like being told to break off a chunk of who you are and flush it down the drain. It seems ludicrous to you, and it probably feels like harassment.

Realize you are more emotionally vulnerable than you were before lupus, perhaps more than you've ever been before. Managing your emerging sensitivity is a learning process that cannot be accomplished overnight. You may make mistakes in the way you respond to comments and suggestions, but that's okay. For now, try to field those frustrating comments one at a time and know that the longer you're on the path to wellness, the better you will become at handling those suggestions that infuriate you.

3) SOME PEOPLE WILL NOT KNOW HOW TO REACT

Some people will be better at dealing with your illness than others. Some won't know what to say or how to say it. When they do ask about lupus, their inquiries sound like accusations. The questions they pose about your job, household chores, or social plans just seem like opportunities to point out your failings. You're struggling enough as it is to make sense of your newly limited abilities. Doesn't their intuition tell them to have the decency not to bring it up all the time?

Others may be silent. In fact, the people whom you expected to understand the most may not appear to be sympathetic at all. Perhaps you'd like them to acknowledge that you're sick in the first place, because from the way they're acting, it seems like they don't believe you really are. They may show very little concern for your situation, interacting with you as if nothing has changed. They don't understand the pain and misery you're forced to live with each day and, therefore, appear to have no compassion.

You're not capable of tackling this disease alone, but if those around you continue to exacerbate the problem, you may have no choice. You spend as much time defending yourself as you do fighting off the effects of the disease. Can't they see the detriment they're causing?

While there are many communicative blunders that can occur in any relationship, the interjection of a third party, in this case a chronic illness, can all but stifle an otherwise normal encounter. It may be impossible for you to fathom the insensitivity or inconsideration that others have toward your bout with lupus. But it may be just as difficult for those around you to make sense of how you're dealing with the disease. Their attitude toward you has changed, and it's up to you to figure out how lupus has affected your relationship. You need to consider the new boundaries that have arisen in order to reopen the lines of communication that have closed.

❝ *Life in general and good relationships with other human beings in particular don't have to be difficult. In fact, if they are, maybe you need to reevaluate your approach.* [2]

During your exploration, you might find it necessary to make significant changes in the way you relate to people (and with whom you relate). You may need to establish a set of ground rules for yourself or for others in order to avoid certain situations. Perhaps you need to separate yourself temporarily from those who are struggling to adapt to your new life with lupus. It may be advantageous for you both to take some time and space to get used to the changes that are occurring.

The steps to better communication

1) PREPARE TO UNDERSTAND

Most people around you don't have lupus, and hopefully, they never will. There-fore, they will never fully comprehend what it's like to have the disease. The more you attempt to explain it, the more frustration you may cause yourself. Without a point of reference, your descriptions of the mental and physical anguish you encounter are futile. Maybe your female friends have experienced swollen fin-gers during pregnancy or perhaps your athletic friends can identify with joint pain or exhaustion. But neither group can ever fully grasp the enormity of having a disease in which: a) symptoms like these can't be attributed to a temporary state of being or a particular activity and b) these ailments may never cease to exist. You could spend a lifetime trying to convey the nature and severity of your pain and suffering in contrast to the symptoms they've experienced, but why waste the time? Let go of your own expectations to be heard and take a break from defend-ing yourself and correcting their misconceptions. Instead of straining to be un-derstood, strive to understand the limited perspective of those around you. Learn to accept the constraints they have of understanding you and your disease. People are always going to try and identify with your situation. How open you are to their attempts will improve your relationships and make communicating about lupus that much easier.

2) PLAN TO BE PATIENT

Because the disease plays a role in almost every relationship you have, your friends and family members will need time to adjust to the intrusion, just as you did. Believe it or not, you may adapt to your limitations before others do. Your physical ailments serve as a constant reminder that you can't do something; your husband, kids, or co-workers don't have that built-in cue. They may need a recap from time to time. Enjoy the fact that you don't look as sick as you are - although I know it's not as great as not looking as old as you are. Instead of taking offense when someone asks you to do something beyond your ability, take a moment to re-educate him or her on your actual limitations. You may need to work together to make their misconceptions match reality.

My sister, for instance, had her own ideas about how little I should be doing during my worst bouts with lupus, and for good reason. She nursed me back to health month after month, taking on the role of caretaker as only an older sister who lives five minutes away could. She was instrumental in my recovery. However, because of her close involvement, she tried to prevent me from engaging in any activity that might flare my disease. That restrictiveness, while well intended, made me feel shackled. The more I tried to test my own limits to maintain my sanity, she was there to try to clip my wings for safety. My only wish is that I could have appreciated her point of view, rather than lashing out and fighting back. Had I exercised more patience and understanding, I would have realized how desperate she was to protect her little sister from the misery I endured. I could have spent less time defending myself and more time collaborating with her. If I had, we might have been able to come up with a plan to restore my health, without sacrificing my dignity or her peace of mind.

3) CONSIDER THE FEELINGS OF OTHERS

A friend of mine suffers from a rare kidney disease and, for far too long, she kept the fact from her two sons. She had convinced herself that, "if nobody else knew about it, it wasn't true." I've had this same thought myself, believing that if no one knew how high my fever was or how swollen my joints were, I could pretend like I was okay. This misconception leads to a second, more damaging fallacy, which is that the only person really suffering at the hand of your active illness is you. To the contrary, the people who love and care about you want you to be well. The sicker you are and the less you take care of yourself, the more distress you cause them. As I mentioned earlier, it was inconsiderate of me to ignore the emotional trauma I caused my sister. Every time I irresponsibly did something that increased my chances of a flare, I indirectly was causing her stress and anxiety. She didn't need that, nor did she deserve it.

I was being unfair to Johnny, too. Almost every aspect of our lives had been affected since my diagnosis: vacations dwindled, social engagements were limited, even our level of intimacy was compromised. Our fun, spontaneous lifestyle was squashed by the effects of lupus. Yet, I was trying to act as if nothing had changed.

I kept denying that I needed to slow down, even when he specifically asked me to do so. I recall one evening when I was decorating the house for Christmas. It was almost 7:00pm, decorations were strewn everywhere and I hadn't taken a nap. I was exhausted, but I didn't want to stop in the middle of my activity. Johnny came downstairs, took one look at my bleary-eyed face and suggested that I stop, take a nap and finish decorating later. I remember shooting him a look that could kill. I was his spunky, independent, fiery wife; why was he suddenly questioning my judgment about when or if I needed to take a nap? I certainly preferred his typical, laissez-faire attitude to his sudden interest in what I should be doing for the good of my health. *Why did he care anyway?* Well, for one, I was already cranky, and my sour disposition would only continue throughout the evening. Two, I would probably need to sleep through dinner, missing an opportunity to spend time with him, much less prepare anything for us to eat. Had I stopped to consider the daily toll my disease took on him, perhaps I would have been more willing to discuss my health and the steps I could take to improve it. As it was, I wasn't even willing to accept his suggestion about an hour's nap!

I had a responsibility to him, my sister, my friends and the rest of my family to be open and honest about my decline in health. I needed to start making good choices for my benefit and theirs. If I had realized the true impact my un-wellness had on others, perhaps I would have taken better care of myself. Life with lupus is not just about you. The sooner you figure that you out, the sooner you can begin to heal - not just for yourself, but out of consideration for others.

4) ASSUME THE BEST, NOT THE WORST

How many times have you been out, looking relatively healthy and un-lupus-like, when you catch a glimpse of someone hobbling along, struggling to put one foot in front of the other? You know exactly how difficult it is for that person to make his/her joints and muscles move the way they're supposed to. Yet no one would ever guess that you have any inkling of what that feeble person is experiencing. And, yet you do, probably better than most. The same principle applies when you assume others couldn't possibly know what you've experienced. Simply because your counterpart doesn't appear to have first-hand experience with your ailments doesn't mean that they don't. I recall walking into Dr. R's office one day to find him hobbling around with the aid of a cane. Assuming he'd experienced some sort of accident since the last time I saw him (merely eight weeks before), I asked him what recently happened to warrant the walking device. He said, surprisingly, that he'd been suffering from arthritis in his hips for years and that he planned to have a hip replacement before the end of the year. A hip replacement? Arthritis? Dr. R? You mean to tell me that he's dealt with arthritic pain and aching joints the whole time I've been under his care? That was a big shock to me, primarily because he never let on that he was in pain. He also never seemed particularly empathetic to the misery I was experiencing. Of course, he treated me to the fullest extent, but I mistook his insensitivity in doing so as indifference, maybe even dubiousness. I figured he couldn't really grasp the kind of pain I was describing.

For instance, during one appointment, he asked me to explain why I was struggling to walk and what made it so difficult to bend my knees. I assumed he was suspicious of the pain and was looking for symptomatic proof that it really existed. Had I known that he was intimately familiar with the pain I experienced, perhaps I would have been less defensive in my response. I probably didn't come across as combative as I felt, but I could have saved myself frustration and annoyance had I not read into the air of uncertainty that he portrayed. Now I know that his questions are nothing more than benign attempts to uncover the source of the pain, so that he can better diagnose the problem.

I ran into a similar experience at work, with a co-worker who was pestering me to complete my quarterly disability paperwork. (For the span of about two years, my doctor and I were required to complete a company-issued health form justifying the need for me to work reduced hours weekly and to adhere to certain job accommodations, all of which my office was willing and able to make.) These forms proved to be a big hassle, for both my doctor and me, but my co-worker was insistent. She was so forceful that I dreaded seeing her in the hall around the time the forms were due. Why was she so relentless month after month? The circumstances always remained the same, but it seemed she needed more detailed particulars and was more ruthless each quarter. After three or four rounds of experiencing what I felt bordered on harassment, I came right out and asked her why this process had to be so laborious and painstaking, for both of us? She explained that it was in my best interests to have my needs explicitly documented so that if anyone in the company questioned my performance, the accommodations, or the nature of my position, she would have proof (and so would I) that the needs were mandatory and deemed necessary. Well, why hadn't she just said so? Here I thought she was forcing me to get more explicit each time because she herself doubted the need for the accommodations. Had I known, I would have been more compliant.

Even more bizarre was that, unbeknownst to me, this same co-worker had suffered the symptoms of drug-induced lupus, which can have overlapping symptoms with SLE. Once she stopped the suspected medication, her symptoms resolved themselves almost immediately. For almost a week (if not more), however, she experienced the joint pain, fever and flu-like symptoms that she saw me struggle with on a daily basis. Thankfully, she was able to counteract the effect of the medication with her doctor's assistance, but through that experience, she had come to an entirely new understanding of the kind of obstacles I encountered. Who would have guessed that the co-worker whom I felt had the least consideration for my situation ended up being best able to relate to me, even if for just a week?

I often wonder why Dr. R and my co-worker chose not to mention their related experiences to me, but I can't blame them. I've been just as unforthcoming at times. As mentioned, any time my sister would suggest that I slow down or lessen my load, I would instantly lash out at her. I never took the time to explain the reasons for my argumentative behavior because I just didn't think she'd ever understand. When she said unrelentingly "Quit your job," I heard, "Throw away everything you've worked so hard to achieve." I didn't think we would ever reach a resolution. But realizing my oversight, I began to explain what a traumatic process it would be for me. Once I verbalized the loss of identity I feared and demonstrated how trivial she was making the decision, we were able to communicate openly and honestly.

Have you experienced similar misunderstandings with those around you? See if any of these sound familiar:

→ THEY SAID:

You should get some rest.
Don't overdo.
Did you take your medication?
You should stay home from work.
You must be really sick today.
I can help you with that.

What did the doctor say?

→ YOU HEARD:

You look pitiful.
I don't trust you.
You must have messed up.
You can't tough it out.
You're complaining a lot.
You appear to be helpless, so I'll just do it for you.
You're incapable of dealing with this on your own.

> TAKE A MINUTE to think about the way you interpret the suggestions of those around you. How are you translating their words? Are you misconstruing the message? Try writing down the phrases that really anger you on one side of a piece of paper. On the other, write down your interpretation. Notice the disparity between the two, and consider the emotional strings that are attached to the words that upset you. Think about different words or phrases that would be less offensive to you, and then share your findings with those around you. They're probably searching for the right words to use, too!

Now that we've considered the more general aspects of communicating with others, let's take a closer look at the reasons we react to people's questions and comments the way that we do. Specifically, let's consider what I like to call, "the dreaded question."

The dreaded question

It seems harmless enough: one simple question, asked innocently by friends and family. You'd think the sting wouldn't be so bad after awhile, considering that those who ask are generally trying to express their care and concern. Yet the moment the words, "How do you feel?" are uttered, a wave of anger and resentment overcome you. You instinctively grit your teeth and roll your eyes, fighting off the temptation to scream, yell, maybe even curse. For reasons we'll get to in a moment, the inquiry feels like the most insulting and annoying question ever posed. Some days, it's so maddening you can't bear to look the asker in the eye. What's worse is that this first question is often followed by, "Are you feeling better than yesterday?", or the worst one of the bunch, "Do you think you'll feel better tomorrow?". The people who ask are simply showing compassion for your situation, so why do these commonplace questions make you cringe?

While the reasons you take offense may be well founded, they're not clearing your path to wellness. Anger and resentment are draining, stifling even, and the less energy you waste on them the better. Very rarely can you or do you need to change other people, but you can change yourself. In order to effect this change, you need to understand why you react the way you do when people ask what you don't want them to. By evaluating your response, you allow yourself to break down the unspoken barriers that reside between you and those around you. You can then prepare yourself to react in a more rational, agreeable manner with this increased level of self-awareness. Regardless of who's right or wrong, you need to be able to approach these conversations more productively, thus rendering your relationships more beneficial. Letting others propel you down the road to wellness will get you there faster.

For those of you stumped by the fact that your naïve questions could ever be misconstrued as hurtful, don't despair. Your simple expressions of concern aren't inherently wrong. But, when posed in the form of a question to someone struggling with a chronic illness, they can cause a surge of emotional heartache and trauma already brewing below the surface. Read on to find out why.

TOP FIVE REASONS YOU HATE THE "DREADED QUESTION"

1) YOU CAN ONLY ANSWER THE SAME QUESTION SO MANY TIMES WITHOUT BECOMING ANNOYED.

Ask anyone struggling with a chronic illness, and they'll tell you that everyone they know asks this very same dreaded question. I still get it, even in my healthy state. After years of fighting it and years of becoming infuriated because yet another person asked me how I was doing, I've learned to focus on people's thoughtfulness rather than the annoyance factor. There's too much love and sincerity attached to these questions to become offended. Obviously, the people who ask do so because they care. No one is deliberately trying to drive you mad. How are they to know that you've been asked that question a dozen times today!

If you come to expect the million-dollar question, you can better prepare yourself for the repetition. Just take the question at face value, rather than dwell on the bevy of thoughts and emotions the question conjures up in your mind. After all, the question itself isn't bad. Check it out. How. Do. You. Feel. Not so terrible, right? If you know you're going to get asked, detach yourself from the emotion of the question, and instead appreciate the fact that someone's asking after you.

2) WHEN YOU RESPOND TRUTHFULLY TO THE QUESTION, PEOPLE REACT POORLY.

Consider this:

→ A percentage of those who ask don't really want to hear a truthful answer; they're just asking to be polite.

→ A percentage of those who ask want to know the truth, but they don't have the time to hear about it right now.

→ A percentage of those who ask want to hear every detail you have to offer and they are offended when you don't tell them.

In regard to the first and second groups of people, don't blame them. Sidestepping your response or reacting in shock when your answer isn't the perfunctory, "Fine, thanks for asking," doesn't mean they don't care about you or how you're feeling. Maybe it's hard for the person to talk about illness, pain, or discomfort. Maybe it's too close to a situation they've been through before. Maybe they're worried that they'll say the wrong thing back. By simply asking the question, they're able to express their concern while possibly avoiding any further involvement. In fact, they've probably asked you this question before, and you've probably answered, "Fine, thanks," the majority of the time. You've actually trained them to anticipate a brief and impersonal response. You've repeatedly chosen not to expound. While that's perfectly normal, the expectation has been set. For you to decide suddenly that today is the day you're going to reveal how you're actually feeling isn't entirely fair.

Now, for those of you who do ask, and don't want any answer other than a "Fine" or an otherwise uninvolved answer, take this advice: don't ask. Choose another line, maybe something declarative like, "I hope you're feeling better today." In this way, you're not soliciting a response that you don't want anyway, nor are you baiting the person you ask. They'll appreciate the thoughtfulness of your declaration, and you can leave it at that.

3) THE PEOPLE YOU THINK SHOULD WANT TO HEAR EVERY DETAIL OF YOUR ANSWER DON'T WANT TO HEAR IT.

Good listeners, that is, individuals who absorb what they're being told and do so supportively, encouragingly and without judgment, are invaluable. My mom falls into this category, and I don't know what I would do without her. Sometimes, though, the people closest to you aren't good listeners, and the people you think should be in this category are not. Don't press the issue. A good listener is never forced into listening. If someone close to you isn't quite ready for a full-blown explanation of how you're *really* feeling, meet them half way. Acknowledge that they've asked, but hold off on the gory details for now. Seek out that good listener of yours – the one who's dying to know the latest in your struggle to be well, and unleash the details on her. Open your mind to friends and co-workers to fill this role; someone not living in the same household as you may be your best bet.

4) YOU'RE TOO SPENT TO ANSWER THE QUESTION RIGHT NOW.

Most of the time, it's easiest to respond to this question with a one-word answer, primarily because you don't have the energy, strength, or brain power to describe in detail how you're feeling. This lethargy is the result of having a chronic illness linked with pain, fatigue and cloudiness. It's okay to try and slide by without going into too much detail. But if you're not going to offer an explanation, you can't expect people to miraculously infer how you're really feeling. Don't assume they know that you truly don't feel well or what you say isn't really what you mean. If you say you're fine, people are going to think you are, guess what, fine. There are those close to you who can read right through your bogus answers (*e.g.* my sister), but it doesn't mean that everyone else can, too. If you don't elaborate, don't be surprised if there isn't an outpouring of concern for your well-being. Remember, with a simple, one-word response, people are taking the cue that there's nothing more to discuss. They're simply respecting your privacy and mirroring your brevity.

5) IT IS AGAINST YOUR NATURE TO TALK ABOUT SUCH DISCOURAGING SUBJECTS LIKE HOW BAD YOU FEEL.

Ah-ha! Now you're getting somewhere. You've arrived at the inner workings of the chronically ill, the traits that keep you from healing, the real opportunities for you to grow. Here it is, in a nutshell: the expectations you have for yourself to appear strong, capable and undaunted are higher than the expectations others have for you. It's easier to put up a good front, convincing others (and yourself) that you're actually not feeling tired and vulnerable than to be honest about how you feel. You believe if you don't talk about the pain, you won't validate the pain. This should make you stronger, but it doesn't. In fact, your denial weighs you down even more. When you don't answer questions truthfully, you are assuming that what you want others to hear - something positive, hopeful, unselfish, and deflective - is what they want to hear, too. That isn't always true or fair, and it certainly isn't healthy.

It took me a long time to admit that my way wasn't always the right way. I thought that because I didn't look sick, maybe I could act like I wasn't sick. I hoped to push my way through the disease, secretly dodging one symptom after another. In appearance, I could at least look normal. Don't we all want to appear normal? In fooling ourselves, however, we're not fooling the disease. In fact, we're fueling its fire. By continually denying how we feel and refusing to own up to the fact that maybe our body isn't working at 100%, we're letting the disease slowly get the best of us. When we shut out those around us by not being honest with ourselves or with them, we give up the opportunity to "share" the pain, not physically, but emotionally. Who couldn't use a hand in shouldering the burden? By admitting that we're "moving a little slower," "feeling a little achy," or down right, "having an awful day," we're breaking down the barriers between ourselves, those who love us and the disease itself.

Clearly, the question, "how are you feeling today?" isn't quite as straightforward as it might first appear. Each one of us, askers and answerers alike, have our own agendas, expectations, and comfort zones in which we operate. Acknowledging these truths should bring us to a new understanding about ourselves and those around us. Doing so enables us to cope with the emotional roller coaster on which we are riding. I firmly believe we can live in harmony with our chronic illness, as long as truth, honesty and self-awareness reside alongside us.

After more than eight years with lupus, I attribute much of my good health and success to my family, friends and co-workers. Without them, I wouldn't have had the courage to make the choices I've made. I've learned that, by embracing others, that is, by sharing my pain, I can wield enough power to conquer lupus a dozen times over. Aren't we lucky we only have to do it once?

CHAPTER 6:
ASK FOR AND
ACCEPT HELP

Having worked the exercises up to this point in the book, you should recognize that neither your identity nor your value as a human being is dependent on what you can accomplish. You're multi-faceted and dynamic. Armed with courage and self-assurance, you're ready to divest yourself of the areas of your life that serve as a constant drain. You want to work smarter, not longer; listen more, talk less; simplify life; not complicate it. Your long, productive future is worth your efforts; you not only want to believe it, you now know it to be true.

You're open to the generosity others have to offer and are eager to start living a better, healthier lifestyle. You know there are lifestyle adjustments to be made, and you're convinced it's time to start making them. But how do you begin to capitalize on the goodwill of those around you? How do you determine which areas of your life need help, and how do you go about asking for it?

We'll make it easy by focusing on two categories of activities: areas of your life where your productivity level is no longer to the level of your liking and areas that cause you stress. Altering your behavior as it relates to either category will undoubtedly change the way you live life with lupus forever.

With any change comes a period of adjustment, and that stage of your journey shouldn't be overlooked. As you begin to eliminate activities, you may experience pangs of remorse or feel as though you are sacrificing more than just an inconsequential part of your daily routine. The activities you're engaged in are important to you, otherwise you wouldn't be doing them. Just as you have in previous exercises, allow yourself a moment to grieve for the loss. At the same time, remind yourself that the accommodations you make are intended to lengthen your life, not hamper it. You are not compromising your quality of life; you are taking steps to improve it.

Remember, too, that there is no one to blame or prevent you from seeking this healthier way of life but you. Whatever commitments you feel are preventing you from making the necessary changes, be it your job, an unhealthy relationship, or a responsibility to care for someone else (an aging parent or children), find a way to let the emotional attachment to those responsibilities go once and for all. This isn't an easy goal, but it is an attainable one. This chapter is designed to help you figure out how to achieve it. In it, you'll learn how to

> → Critically evaluate your activity levels at both work and home
> → Find strategic ways to cut back on your activities in such a way that empowers rather than undermines you
> → Make practical alterations to even the most routine of activities

The tips and suggestions made in the following pages take into consideration the fact that you still have a busy, fulfilling life to lead. They'll allow you to still get done what you need to, but in a healthier, more balanced manner. The adjustments you make will adapt your lifestyle to your new goal of living well, enabling you to maintain a healthier outlook for years to come.

Every day for the rest of your life, you'll be making the choice to live well. You're fully capable of making that right choice; don't just think you are, know you are.

❝ *It isn't so important what disease the patient has as what kind of patient has the disease.* [1]

Believe that you have the knowledge, wisdom and experience necessary to make these critical decisions. You may see nothing but obstacles in your path, a roadway littered with responsibility and commitment. But, those blockades are nothing compared to the mental roadblocks you've already hurdled in your struggle with lupus. Now it's time to put that mental resolve (and ingenuity) to good use.

Guidelines for letting go

Making the decision to start letting go is a big one. It's a huge step toward under-standing, coping with and conquering your disease. Visions of a pain-free, ful-filling life should be clearer than they were before. If they are, consider yourself within close range of your objective. Before we get into the logistics of making the changes that accompany this decision, there are three minor points that should be addressed so you can permanently live well with your disease:

1) DISTINGUISH BETWEEN VOLUNTARY AND INVOLUNTARY DECISIONS

Picture the following scenario:

You've had a terrible day. You dragged your aching body into the office early, worked through lunch and dealt with one irate client after another. You just spent the last hour rehashing their complaints to your boss, making you late for your evening's agenda of dinner with out-of-town friends. Your head is pounding, your joints are throbbing, and you can feel painful swelling beginning to take shape. Physically, you want to collapse on the floor of your office and wake up in three days. Instead, you mentally prepare to wear your pain-free "game face" for the evening. As you're frantically heading out of the office, your husband calls to let you know that something's come up and your friends aren't going to be able to make it tonight. He tells you to just head for home. He's ordered take-out for the two of you, and it will be ready and waiting when you get there. Relieved that the only thing you're destined for tonight is a relaxing, restful evening at home, you tidy up your desk and head home.

Caught a break, didn't you? You got lucky, and you know it. You were able to dodge yet another evening of pain, suffering, and overdoing, although the majority of your day wasn't very pleasant.

If this was catching a break, think for a moment what *taking* a break would have in-volved. What would have happened if you had: evaluated whether an extra hour of sleep would have been more beneficial than rushing in to get an early start at the office, taken a break for a nutritious lunch, asked your boss if you could fill him in first thing in the following morning, and/or voluntarily canceled your dinner plans? It would have been an entirely different kind of day. It might have been a lot less painful and lot more manageable.

Acknowledging the difference between getting a break from your hectic, demanding lifestyle and taking one comes down to one simple thing: you. Every day, you have the power to decide how painful the day is going to be. I know you can't control lupus, but you can control your willingness to adapt to it.

For example, although grabbing a catnap when you're tired might not sound daunting, consider that the act of sleeping isn't the difficult part. It's allowing yourself the time to get the extra rest in the first place. Take a weekend when you find yourself with an hour to spare. Would you voluntarily take a nap? No, you'd rather catch up on errands or projects around the house. However, what if someone in your family insisted that you take an hour to rest and relax? What if they went so far as to dim the lights, pull the shades in your bedroom and turn down the sheets on your bed? What if they ushered you under the covers and tucked you in nice and tight so that you felt warm and cozy? Do you think you could manage a wink or two? I bet you could.

Furthermore, if someone in your family insisted on doing the laundry or vacuuming, could you comply? And, what if your boss prohibited you from taking on any additional projects at work? Could you handle it? Probably so. Situations like these are no-brainers. But voluntarily doing so? That's a different story. Once you realize how much you're relying on those involuntary moments to save you from yourself, you can begin to willfully (and of your own accord) make those decisions for yourself. You must enable yourself to make smart, responsible, deliberate decisions and allow yourself to start letting go, *voluntarily*.

2) GIVE YOURSELF PERMISSION

I've asked you to grieve for yourself and for the abilities you've lost due to the limitations of your disease. I also suggested that you embrace others and allow them to be involved in your recovery. Now, marry the two together by asking for help in areas where you need it and willingly accept it.

For almost every task you have on your to-do list, there is probably an easier, more efficient way of tackling it. That method, of course, most likely involves employing the help of someone else. This approach may not be your first inclination. Nor does it necessarily satisfy your ego or appeal to your "do it yourself" nature. But if you can put those things aside, the everyday decisions you face don't have to be accompanied with pain or difficulty. Choosing to use a caterer (or ordering take-out) for a dinner party rather than slaving over the stove yourself could be the best decision you make all day. Ordering a gift online rather than traipsing out to the mall could save you loads of time and energy. Regardless of the task, believe that you (and the future of your health) are worth the extra expense or forethought to make life just a little more tolerable.

When I consider the pain and anxiety that going to the grocery store used to cause me, I realize how unfair I was being to my body. Just contemplating the thought of walking those tile floors and hauling the groceries from the cart to the car and then into the house was enough to send me into a panic attack. Usually I was so fatigued by the time I'd completed my mission, all I could do was collapse into bed before putting the groceries away. I certainly could have relinquished the chore to my husband or a friend. Yet, the thought of sending someone else to do the job seemed like an even bigger waste of time and frustration. I knew which brands to buy, was familiar with the store's layout, and I felt silly pawning off such a simple task.

Because the effects of my shopping trip would eventually subside, I convinced myself that it was worth the trouble. But did they really? Simple activities like grocery shopping were actually causing the majority of my difficulty. Why did I continue to waste my precious time and limited energy on something as mundane as picking up groceries? *There must be a better way to get the job done.* So I started exploring my alternatives. I could ask a friend or delegate the task to Johnny, but that would just raise questions and create more work for me. How about ordering my groceries online and having them delivered? Wasn't that only for the sick and homebound, and wasn't there a delivery fee involved? Wouldn't I be embarrassed when the delivery person showed up to the house of a seemingly able-bodied 30-year old? How could I justify spending the extra money just to save myself the hassle? Would I still be able to get all of the products I needed? Would they pick out the best produce? Would they arrive when I needed them to?

My skepticism almost got the best of me, but because I'd promised myself to look into alternative options, I followed through on my research. As it turned out, the delivery service in my area carried almost all of my favorites products. The turn-around time for delivery could be as soon as the following day, and the steep delivery fee I imagined was a mere $6 if I ordered $100 worth of groceries.

Wasn't my health worth a measly $6 a week? In fact, what if I added lunchmeat to my grocery order and made a sandwich one day a week instead of ordering out from the deli. Wouldn't I make back my $6? What's more, I could order my groceries any time of day or night. I could be resting in bed, grab the laptop and order my groceries, right there from my bed! And, to think that my days of wobbly shopping carts and heavy bags of dog food or water bottles might be over. It brings me relief just thinking about it.

Are you, too, holding out on yourself, maybe for as little as $6? Give yourself permission to take advantage of the services available to you, rather than experience the unnecessary hassle, pain and suffering that could be eliminated from the day. Why not? You are worth it!

3) ALTER YOUR PERSPECTIVE

It's natural for you to see things from a certain point of view – it makes you who you are. But, remember, you're endeavoring to reconfigure the way you think, feel and live. In doing so, you're bound to need a slightly broader outlook than the one you currently have.

This is different from simply listening to the opinions of others. Now I'm asking you to seek out another perspective voluntarily in order to enlighten yourself. You may not agree with the alternate line of thinking, but at least you can compare it with your original approach. Even if the experience simply strengthens your convictions about your own perspective, you'll have learned something along the way.

Remember how I said my sister used to hound me to quit my job? One summer when I was really struggling with lupus, she became particularly insistent that I do something to start helping my situation. The arguments that ensued took a toll on our relationship for the rest of the summer, and we had tension and tears almost every time we spoke. She couldn't understand my reluctance to make a change at work. I wasn't prepared to make such a drastic change in my life. My situation was complicated, and it would take time to come up with the right solution. She would just have to deal with it.

In my defense, I knew the long hours and demanding work schedule contributed to my health problems. I'd been keeping my chronic control spreadsheet long enough to see the correlation. I knew that my driven personality needed to be tempered in order to get better, but I was having difficulty acting upon that realization. I considered talking to my boss about reducing the number of hours I worked, per a standing offer he'd made months earlier, but I wasn't convinced that more idle time would have a positive effect on my illness. In fact, I thought it actually might be worse to be stuck at home without anything to take my mind off of lupus. After further contemplation, I concluded that I really didn't want to reduce our household income, lose the level of responsibility I'd worked hard to attain, or put the company in an awkward or compromising position. My job as a manager wasn't an expendable position. How could I just start working less? It wasn't typical, nor was it the way I wanted to conduct myself at work.

Katie was exasperated by my inaction, so she suggested I accompany her to her next therapy appointment. She said it might help her cope with my inability to act, while giving me some professional insight into my situation. If it accomplished these objectives and alleviated the strain between us, it would be well worth the time and effort. In the end, I went willingly.

We went to the appointment and, after twenty minutes of chitchat, the therapist asked me a couple of questions about how the stress of my job related to my illness. I admitted that the two were connected, but I wasn't convinced that working a reduced workweek was the right thing for me to do. There were a lot of things to consider, and I wasn't sure I was prepared for the change in lifestyle. Her response was a very simple, noncommittal, "I guess you could at least try it and see how it goes. If it doesn't work out, you don't have to keep doing it." She said this completely void of emotion, opinion, or hidden agenda, which I loved. For the first time, it seemed as though attempting to work less might be a very practical, non-threatening option to pursue. It didn't have to be a permanent change, and I liked the open-endedness of the decision. The way she'd posed the offer, I really couldn't say anything but, "I guess I could try it." To this day, I give my sister credit for not shouting out "Hallelujah" or some other gleeful response. She just nodded her head, smiled, and then carried on with the rest of the appointment.

Within a few days of the meeting with the therapist, I approached the director of human resources at my company with the proposal. She immediately agreed, suggesting I reduce my workday from nine hours to six and work one day from home. The conversation took all of ten minutes. She and my boss both knew I had been struggling to keep up, and they were supportive of any solution that might improve my health.

In the end, this decision I'd agonized over turned out to be one of the best changes I made. Had my sister not persisted, and had I not agreed to go to the appointment, I don't know where I would be today!

The next time I found myself struggling with a similar decision, I jumped at the opportunity to broaden my outlook and get another perspective. As I contemplated making another job change, this time to a part-time position working from home, I thought about the articles in almost every lupus-related health magazine devoted to issues about finding the balance between work and a healthy lifestyle. In the past, I avoided reading those magazines because I felt some of the firsthand accounts were too depressing. The stories describing personal bouts of strife and difficulty caused by the disease upset me quite a bit. Thus, I chose to forgo them altogether.

One day, though, I found myself at the doctor's office, and although I hadn't read one of those magazines in years, I picked one up. I thought if ever there was a time when I needed a little help working through my issues with lupus, it was now. I flipped open the magazine to the first page and there, in the bottom corner, was a small paragraph from a reader, thanking the publication for a recent story. In this short, 3-line note, the reader declared that she recently had switched from a full-time, demanding job to a part-time, work-from-home position and that it had lessened her disease activity. For the first time in years, she was feeling good, had energy and was happy. Right then and there, I decided that, if this random woman quoted in the magazine could downshift her life and make it better, so could I.

It's easy to convince yourself that you have all the answers. And yes, your way may be the best way to proceed. But once you admit that a different take on life with lupus might be just what you need, life gets a whole lot easier. You won't have to try so hard to come up with the perfect solution on your own. You'll find value in listening and considering what others think and feel and you'll benefit from letting them help you solve your problems. You should appreciate that someone else is willing to lead you to the answers you seek, taking the pressure off your already burdened shoulders.

> " *Precious Lord, take my hand*
> *–Lead me on, let me stand*
> *I'm tired, I'm weak, I'm lone*
> *–Through the storm, through the night*
> *Lead me on to the light*
> *–Take my hand precious*
> *Lord, lead me home.* [2]

Evaluating your productivity

Begin by thinking about how you define "You." How do you view yourself with and without lupus? What personality traits are most apparent? Have those changed since your diagnosis? When I asked myself these questions, I saw myself as follows: outgoing, a perfectionist, a good manager and well-organized. So were these attributes still applicable in my current state of illness?

First, I had to admit that I wasn't quite as gregarious as I used to be. Yes, I was amicable, but I just didn't have the energy to be extroverted anymore. I thought of the last few dinner parties I'd attended. At each one, I sat quietly in a corner without really participating, desperately trying to make it through the evening without succumbing to fatigue, pain, or both.

Second, my desire for perfection was still present, but my standards weren't what they once were. They couldn't be, as my body was no longer capable of enduring the pressure.

And with my most recent health problems and reduced work schedule, was I flourishing in my career? I was still working, but my performance wasn't stellar or consistent. Was I living up to the expectations I had (or my company had) of a hands-on, successful manager or employee?

I needed to acknowledge that a) I wasn't operating at full capacity at home or at work, b) I was more effective when I was healthy, and c) I wasn't performing any task better or faster than someone else could. Acknowledging the truth in each of these statements was difficult, but I grappled with the third one the most. Wasn't I the only one who could do my job as I did? Wouldn't the household fall apart if I stopped taking charge? As much as I wanted to believe the answers to these questions were true, I couldn't deny the reality of the situation. Although I was making significant contributions, I wasn't indispensable.

A friend of mine in the leadership training arena opens each of his training sessions with the following statement:

> **"** *Please turn off all cell phones and pagers. If you happen to subscribe to the myth of indispensability, then at least switch your phone to the vibrate position.*[3]

While this statement made me chuckle the first time I heard it, it reminded me that if I took a break from my busy lifestyle, life would still go on. In fact, I could make *more* of an impact if I took time off to get healthy. I could reduce the tasks I was struggling to accomplish and instead focus on just a few that I knew I could do well, despite my disease. I had never been content at being second best, so wouldn't life be more enjoyable if I was actually succeeding at it?

If you haven't experienced any change in performance up to this point, great. But now is as good of a time as any to evaluate what activities might aggravate your disease in the future. It's better to preempt the potential fallout than allow your job performance to slip or your duties at home to suffer. Of course, if your level of productivity has been compromised, finding the motivation to modify your behavior shouldn't be difficult. You know the consequences of your actions; now it's time to do something about it.

TO START PARING DOWN, pinpoint a couple of areas of your life that you know aren't going very well. In this particular exercise, I don't want you to brainstorm on the activities that you think you are performing well. You may be underestimating what you can still do and your limited thinking might dissuade you from completing the exercise. Instead, think of two or three activities in which you are engaged where you're disappointed in your performance. By revising just a few things on your schedule, dropping an extra-curricular activity, canceling a couple of events on your social calendar or reducing your responsibilities at work, you'll free up time to rest and reenergize, making you feel more alive and engaged than before. You may even have the energy to endeavor upon other activities you never thought possible, those that fulfill without jeopardizing your health. I promise you: living well, despite your disease, will not be a disappointing venture.

IN THE WORKPLACE

My own experience in modifying my work schedule couldn't have been better. The flexibility my company gave me was phenomenal, particularly as I struggled to balance my work responsibilities with the disease limitations. When I returned to work after being out for a month with my first flare, my supervisor and I agreed I should start with partial days and then work up to full-time. We agreed that I would come in around 9:00am and leave no later than 1:00 or 2:00pm. But I couldn't force myself to leave. When he saw me struggling to do so, he suggested I come in at noon or 1:00pm and work through the end of the day instead. He knew I didn't have the discipline to put my health first, so he stepped in to make it happen. Every subsequent supervisor demonstrated that same level of consideration. I often was reminded via email or voicemail not to work too hard and to take the time I needed to get well. Despite my frequent doctor's appointments, sick days, late starts, early finishes and days worked from home, the company's sympathetic nature made a huge difference in my ability to cope at work.

But I must admit the situation wasn't without effort on my part. For instance, when I asked for shortened workdays, I made sure that the hours I put in were worthy of a full day's worth of work. I spent little time socializing while in the office. I knew my work schedule was an exception to the rule, and I was committed to making sure my company didn't regret the liberty they were extending to me. Also, I took as few sick days as possible, never taking advantage of the policy or abusing the flexibility I was given. I never once took a day when I wasn't stuck in bed, so my supervisors knew that when I called in, I was sick. Additionally, as candid and upfront as I was about what I wasn't able to take on, I was even more enthusiastic and forthcoming about what I *could* do. Eventually, I researched the company's needs and plans for the future, and created a work-from-home position specifically designed to meet one of their growing demands. I was intimately familiar with the issues that needed to be addressed and presented a solution to make sure it was met.

One of the biggest compliments I received came from the president and owner of the company, on one of my final days of work. I was expressing my gratitude for all of the accommodations he and his staff had made for me over the years, and he said to the contrary, he wanted to thank me for all of my years of service. From his point of view, it wasn't my requests for special treatment that stood out; it was the solution-oriented approach I put forth every step of the way. I was a good employee, a respected and trusted part of the team, and the company was as good to me as I was to them.

What did I learn from my experiences at work, which in turn helped me adjust my commitments at home? I learned that honesty, initiative, and solution-oriented thinking will get you where you need to go – hopefully on the path to living well. Let's take a closer look at each of these attributes:

1) Be upfront: I find it best to be as honest with as many people as possible about the disease, its limitations, and requirements (medication, rest, etc.). I respect those of you who have chosen, for whatever reason, to keep the matter of your disease quiet at work or outside of your immediate circle of friends. I can speak only to the warm reception I experienced from co-workers, friends and acquaintances. Of course, there were always a few people who couldn't quite grasp why I was missing work or friends who didn't understand why I couldn't make a weekend getaway. But the majority of those around me appreciated being involved in my life with lupus.

I couldn't have negotiated my disease alone. It was invaluable to collaborate and brainstorm with those around me, particularly about the changes I needed to institute at work and at home. I valued their support and constantly needed their understanding. In fact, if my performance at work did slip, it was easier to manage since those around me knew that I had lupus. It was always a big relief not to have to cover for my disease. The encouragement you receive will pleasantly surprise you.

A woman from my lupus group shared a story that echoes this sentiment. She was working as a contractor for a company that recently placed her on a long-term project working onsite with a client. The company she worked for was well aware of her disease, but they had requested that she not share that information with the client. She agreed, but within a few months of starting her assignment, it was apparent that her workload and long, demanding hours with this new client were not going to jibe with her health needs. She knew the situation easily could be resolved if she shared knowledge of her health situation with the client, but her parent company continued to insist on her secrecy.

She wasn't asking for much – simply to work no more than eight hours a day with no expectation for overtime – and knew it was in everyone's best interest to reveal her condition. She finally insisted that her company notify the client on her behalf. They finally acquiesced, and the client was very accepting of the nominal changes in her work schedule. In fact, they were thrilled to have been apprised of the entire situation. She resumed a more normal work schedule, which consequently lessened her disease activity.

Being upfront can also apply at home or in your social circles. If making your weekly girls' night out is too much for you, invite the girls over for pizza or a movie. You'll be able to enjoy their company while not overexerting yourself. They'll be happy you're taking care of yourself and enlisting them to take part in your efforts.

2) Take the initiative: I've never been particularly shy or patient, so addressing issues quickly and forcefully came naturally. In fact, my proactivity at work proved to be a helpful trait to which my employer responded favorably.

Thankfully, they never had to approach me about my lack of performance or slip in productivity because at each juncture, I addressed the issue first. For example, I approached them about changing my workload; I later suggested that I wasn't living up to the expectations of the job; and I finally decided when and how I needed to accommodate the disease. It saved them from having to craft a diplomatic approach to an already sensitive subject. I'm not naïve to the fact that, if the situation had become too unreasonable, they would have been forced to address the issue. I felt good about the changes I was making because I was the one instigating the adjustment, not someone else. To initiate change is both empowering and rewarding, and it's usually easier than to doing so at the request of another.

Just because you've lost some mobility doesn't mean you've lost all sense of leadership or ingenuity. You still have your brainpower; now you just have to start using it. It's your responsibility to show others how to work around your limitations and how they can help in the process.

3) Present solutions: As a project manager in the television post-production industry, solving problems was an everyday occurrence. It was an expected part of the position, and the term "Fix it in Post" wasn't coined without reason. The quick turnaround projects, outrageous client demands, or last minute details required that I act as a constant troubleshooter for my clients and for the company as a whole.

The problems I encountered almost always required the expertise of a trained technical professional: a late-night project needed a creative artist to stay late or come in early, a weekend film shoot required a cameraperson, or a last-minute satellite feed needed a technician in order to make an airdate. While I was ultimately responsible for handling these issues, I couldn't resolve them on my own. I needed help, so I learned to act quickly and authoritatively. Things worked out for me most of the time, primarily because I was surrounded by people who cared about their jobs and the clients we served. But also, instead of dwelling on a problem, the first thing I did was work toward a solution. Learning to involve others who could actually solve those problems was paramount.

I became very good at crisis management. I kept cool under pressure and got the job done time and again. In fact, I was often the person others came to in the company when a problem arose. I embraced the challenge each time and tried to teach others that I was only as good as the people who were willing to perform the work. It always felt good to provide a service in which I could see tangible results, work as a team and truly make a difference in the company.

However, when I started to falter due to the symptoms of lupus, I struggled with my new limitations. I suddenly found it difficult to think as quickly or rationally as I used to. I wasn't able to dash through the facility to address last minute demands or abate crises. I wanted to prove to myself and everyone else that lupus wasn't going to hold me back, so I desperately tried to assert myself. I wanted to show the team that I still could do my part, despite my illness. The more I tried to do this, the fewer tasks I delegated. Thus, the more I worked, the sicker I became. Desperate for an objective viewpoint, I candidly asked my team how I might improve the situation. They all agreed that I needed to take on less and give away more. They didn't want me to be unwell, and they could see that if I allowed them to pick up the slack, I would not only get better, but the tasks could be done more efficiently and effectively. All I needed was to pass off the work and then allow them to do their jobs. It was problem solving at its most basic level.

As I learned, you can't let your own personal agenda or hang-ups get in the way of your willingness to create solutions, particularly if they're related to your illness. You may feel like you don't want to let go of a certain aspect of your work or home life. You may convince yourself that holding on is still the best approach. But realize the heroics that are involved when you create a better solution than the meager one you're currently able to offer. Backing down from a task doesn't always equate to shirking responsibility, particularly if you're doing so to get better results. This might not be feasible or acceptable, depending on your job, but if it is, seize the opportunity to set an example for those around you. You'll be taking steps to improve the state of your own health, making it acceptable for them to do the same. What a strong message for anyone in a supervisory position to convey.

Eliminating stress

Many stressful situations you encounter are unavoidable. You can't always make the stress of a job, a relationship, or a disease magically disappear, but you can strive to minimize the effect those issues have on your life. While everyone manages stress differently and has their own threshold for how much they can handle, stress is a commonly suspected trigger for lupus[4]. Therefore, the impact it has on your health cannot be taken lightly. Working to eliminate it from your life will have a lasting impression on your overall health and wellness.

When I was still working, two co-workers caused me more stress than the rest of my co-workers combined. Since working with them was unavoidable, I had to devise a way to channel that stress so that my health wouldn't be affected. Remember, I landed myself in the emergency room after a particularly stressful workweek, so I knew I needed to get these situations under control.

After months of trying to figure out how to handle my interactions with them, here's what I tried:

1) I tried to be less sensitive. I concentrated on dismissing their off-handed, hurtful comments rather than taking them personally. I accepted that I was just going to have to learn to live with certain aspects of their personalities. (Acknowledging what you cannot control is just as important as changing what you can.)

2) When I needed to consult with them on an issue, I prepared ahead of time so that I didn't waste their time or mine. I anticipated their questions and concerns so that I wouldn't be caught off guard and our interaction could be short and sweet.

3) When tension arose that was out of my control, I consulted my supervisor. Letting him know (and having him reassure me that they were challenging employees, indeed) made me feel a lot better.

The essence of what I was doing is summarized below, in these three stress-eliminating guidelines that can be applied to many situations:

→ **Set boundaries for yourself**
→ **Use your time wisely**
→ **Get help when you need it**

These are all tall orders for do-it-yourselfers like us, but if I can do it, so can you!

1) SET BOUNDARIES

In 2003, when Kraft Food Inc.'s Nabisco group was brainstorming about new forms of dieting and healthy products, they asked online participants what the words "diet food" represented to them and how they made choices when they snacked. Kraft learned that customers didn't feel they needed to deprive themselves or diet per se – what they really wanted was the ability to control how much they ate. Kraft obliged with 100 Calorie Packs, a line of small, one-person bags of Oreos and Ritz crackers. The results were stunning: In 2005, that product line racked up $100 million in sales.[5] People loved the built-in self-control that accompanied the little snack packs by eliminating the need for willpower.

Example: *naps*

I quite often find myself "dieting" in other aspects of my life, invoking boundaries for myself so that I don't have to decide how much activity, sleep, or stress is enough for one day. A few years into my struggle with lupus, it became apparent that about six or seven hours into each day, I completely lost my momentum. I hit a wall, and after that, I was useless. It was a point at which no amount of sugar, caffeine, or adrenaline could help. I was just too exhausted to do anything. If I was still awake, I walked around in a zombie-like state, pushing myself to function on empty. It was as if the last half of the day wasn't mine anymore; it was lost to fatigue, claimed without recourse. Not only did I lose those hours when I passed my point of total exhaustion, the hour or two before hitting this proverbial "wall" were futile, too. The last scraps of time before I totally lost it were spent fighting off the exhaustion while trying to accomplish the final tasks.

After much deliberation, I convinced myself that if I napped for a couple of hours in the middle of each day, early enough to fend off the "wall" yet late enough not to interfere with the most basic of daily activities, I wouldn't be losing, but gaining time. As long as I got in two hours of sleep sometime around 5:00pm, I would be recharged enough to have a full evening ahead, restocked with energy, stamina, and clarity. A two-hour sacrifice seemed like a small price to pay to make each evening bearable again.

For a while, I treated my nap as an occasional occurrence, but I realized I didn't have the willpower to nap when I needed to. I was too distracted by to-do lists and other things. I needed to set up a constraint for myself so that I couldn't talk myself out of resting each day. Thus, I made it a mandatory part of each afternoon, whether or not I thought I wanted/needed a nap. (Oh, I kicked, screamed, and threw tantrums about going to bed in the beginning.) But, most days, I slept for a solid two hours or even more. It was obvious my body was exhausted (which is probably why I was so cranky to begin with), but I still struggled to force myself into bed each day.

Today, however, my nap is a welcomed part of my daily ritual. I no longer quarrel with myself as I'm lying in bed, swearing that I don't really need to rest. Instead, I look forward to the moment when I can shut my eyes and regroup, confident in the positive result.

Example: *travel*

I've set similar boundaries when it comes to vacations and traveling. Johnny and I learned the hard way that my body doesn't recover from travel packed too closely together. At first, we tried to just be more conscious of our planning, but I wasn't disciplined enough to stick with it. I was always trying to fit in a weekend trip here and there. Now we make it a rule never to set up back-to-back travel weekends and, for a while, we limited ourselves to only one trip per month. Boundaries like these took the guesswork, deliberation, and debate out of the whole planning process, almost guaranteeing that I'd be healthy enough to enjoy the trip from start to finish.

Traveling in general can be a stressful time, but following these guidelines can help you enjoy yourself, each time you hit the road:

MAKE RELAXING A PRIORITY: If your travel plans focus on sightseeing, don't plan a trip chock full of activities. Remember that it's a time of respite. When you arrive at a destination, take a moment to relax and get your bearings. You'll be much better company (and enjoy the festivities to come) if you're well adjusted. Resist the urge to dash about marking items off of your list of must-sees. Instead, set out on a nice, leisurely stroll. If you stop along the way for requisite pictures and snacks, you'll be able to soak up your vacation spot just as much as if you had your nose buried in a sightseeing book. If there is an activity that you definitely want to fit in, allow for plenty of down time before and after the excursion, including time for a sufficient nap. Even if you're on a vacation where the primary goal is to relax, be sure the hours spent "relaxing" don't replace valuable sleep time. Just because you're on vacation doesn't mean that you should allow your health to slip away from you.

Sometimes the actual travel day makes napping a challenge. Therefore, plan for rest time on both ends of the trip. I used to fool myself into thinking that the two or three-hour plane ride (or more) was a sufficient rest. But ending up in a mini-flare each time I flew demonstrated how mistaken I was. Allowing for a little extra rest time is worth the trouble.

DON'T HESITATE TO ASK: Request an early check-in or a late checkout. You'd be surprised how accommodating hotels can be when you say that you have a medical necessity to rest. In fact, one time, I was traveling with my sister and my then 1-year old niece, and my sister called to ask for an early check-in so that my niece could take a nap. When the front desk person didn't seem to be able to help us out, we mentioned the fact that I also needed to take a nap, due to medical necessity and a condition called Systemic Lupus Erythematosus. Immediately, the attendant was able to get us a room. I don't abuse the lupus card, but I am assertive about making sure I take care of myself. There is no need to spoil an entire day (or two) of vacation because I am too embarrassed or shy to talk about my disease!

DOUBLE-CHECK YOUR MEDICATIONS: Just like me, you'd be a mess without your medications and stressed at the consequences of missing a couple of doses. Therefore, always check to make sure you have enough pills to get you through an entire trip and possibly some extras in case of a travel delay.

Also, carry your medicine bag with you for safekeeping, rather than checking it in your baggage. You may get quizzical looks in the security line because you may have a lot of prescriptions. But, in that case, keep a copy of your prescription description (from the drugstore) with you so that you have documentation to show that the pills are indeed prescribed to you. The only exception I made to carrying my drugs on board with me was when I was taking daily injections during my pregnancy. I could have carried the syringes through security, but I needed a newly issued letter from my doctor each time I flew. I preferred to avoid the has-sle, but you may decide that you're more comfortable having the medicines with you at all times, especially if they must be chilled or kept at a specific temperature. Check with the airlines to find out current requirements.

KEEP THE ESSENTIALS PACKED: Keep a second set of the following in your suitcase, rather packing them each time you travel: a hat with a wide brim, a bag of medical supplies (aspirin, bandages, cold/flu medication), sunscreen and travel-size toiletries (like shampoo, conditioner, etc.).

The hat and sunscreen will obviously help when you're in a sunny location and can't seem to find the shade. The medical supplies are for all of the unforeseen issues that crop up with lupus. We're so prone to other health issues that it's nice to have generic, back-up medication on hand. Be sure that all are safe to take in conjunc-tion with your prescriptions. And the toiletries just make packing that much less stressful. The fewer items you have to throw in a bag each time, the better.

I also try and pack the evening before we leave, just so I'm not running around the day I travel. The "day of" is exhausting enough - so eliminate as much stress as possible.

2) USE YOUR TIME WISELY

Value your precious time and energy by spending them on things that deserve your efforts, not those that don't. Only you can determine how your time should be spent, but beware of falling into your old habits. Tackling every single item on your to-do list, including inconsequential "musts", is not good time manage-ment. As you pick and choose the best way to spend your time, don't lose sleep over the things that you simply can't get done. Instead, brainstorm how to do them in some other fashion, putting your brainpower to good use.

If weeding your unsightly garden is important to you, but you just don't have the time or energy to tackle it, hire a gardener or a neighbor kid who wants to earn a few dollars to weed. If the condition of your house is driving you crazy, and you're too spent, hire someone to clean it for you, even if it's not as often as you'd pre-fer. There's no shame in outsourcing, and you should save your time and energy for things that you'd rather be doing or that demand your expertise. I know that outsourcing costs money. But if, for example, hiring a catering service or buying a few pre-made appetizers from a grocery store enables you to throw a party when you wouldn't be able to otherwise, go for it. Money is a consideration, but there are plenty of cost-effective ways to circumvent your limitations. After all, enjoying life is much more important.

Time management also refers to making more efficient use of your time when undertaking projects or in dealing with others. As I mentioned, even though it meant being less social at the office, I chose to limit my chat time with co-workers after I reduced my work hours. Eliminating just a few minutes here and there let me get more done in less time. You can also be more prepared for meetings and appointments in an effort to render them as effective (and as short) as possible. Grouping tasks is another way to save time (and energy) when you're running around the office or catching up on errands. If you're getting up, make the most of your outing by multi-tasking.

Making good use of the time when you lie awake at night is even important. I used to complain to my sister about the sleeplessness I experienced due to my high doses of prednisone. She suggested that if I found myself wide-awake, even in the middle of the night, I should make that time productive. The insomniac effects of prednisone are infamous, so unless you can go back to sleep in about twenty minutes or less, use your time more wisely. Otherwise, you'll drive yourself crazy staring at the ceiling, or even worse, your partner who is sleeping soundly.

What can you do in the middle of the night when you're wide-awake? Put your frustrations down on paper; read a book; watch a thirty-minute program on television; take a bath or shower; order your groceries online; or grab a snack. If you choose to watch television, set a time limit for yourself (a boundary) so that you're not up longer than you need to be. And, if you choose a snack, just choose wisely. Maybe make it a 100-calorie snack pack!

One night when I was wide-awake from about 4:00 to 6:00am, I wrote two full pages of notes about how frustrated I was with lupus and my insomnia. When I went to re-read the notes I had written that next morning, I saw that the pen I'd used was completely out of ink. Not one word was visible on the page! Of course I could have done some investigative work and analyzed the imprint of the pages in order to decipher the words I'd written, but it wasn't worth it. I was probably better off not reading my angst-ridden treatise, and the cathartic writing exercise had served its purpose. It had cleared my head enough so that I eventually went back to sleep.

3) GET HELP

While obtaining help from those around you crosses into the realm of using your time wisely (by choosing to let others do for you what you cannot, should not, or would be better off not doing), asking for assistance deserves it's own category. There are many ways you can simplify your life, options you may have never even considered. When I made a concerted effort to start streamlining my taxing life, I was amazed at all of the little ways in which I could get help. Many were readily available to me; I just wasn't taking advantage of them. I must have been too proud, stubborn, or oblivious to do so. But once I opened myself up to the prospect, I realized that no one but me thought twice about it! No one kept track of the times I enlisted the help of the bagger at the grocery store to get my heavy load from my cart to the car, and no one scoffed when I bought a couple of those jumbo pill boxes with the days of the week on it. For all too long, I resisted doing either of these simple things because I was too embarrassed. But once I got over my own hang-up of not wanting to appear needy, helpless, or incompetent, life got so much simpler. I had had this burning desire not to appear sick, but you know what? I was sick. Once I stopped fooling myself and started thinking of ways to make concessions, I actually started to feel a whole lot better.

ENLISTING HELP
- *Hire a cleaning service*
- *Order your groceries online and have them delivered*
- *Outsource yard work*
- *Accept meals from organizations catering to the sick or homebound*
- *Mail-order your prescriptions*
- *Order gifts online and have them shipped to the recipient directly*
- *Have gifts professionally gift-wrapped — save your swollen fingers the trouble*
- *Hire a caterer when you host a party*
- *Bring a side dish from your favorite restaurant to your next potluck dinner, or buy pre-made dishes from the grocery store*
- *Pull into the full-serve gas pump every once in awhile to give yourself a break*
- *Say "Yes" when the attendant at the grocery store asks, "Need help outside?"*

• *Ask the store clerk to help you with hard-to-unwrap items (e.g. CD's and DVD's, anything with a twist-off cap) immediately after you've purchased them, if no one is at home to help you*
• *Hire someone to walk/groom/care for your pets*
• *Hire a handy man to help with everything and anything around the house*
• *Ask your grocery store deli or bakery to slice, cut, or pre-package items so that you don't have to*
• *Use a dry cleaning service that picks up and delivers*
• *Use the skycap service at the airport or a bellman at a hotel to handle your luggage*
• *Let someone help you when assistance is offered — each and every time*

HELPING YOURSELF

• *Schedule doctors appointments or errands during your most mobile, agile time of the day or week*
• *Switch your wardrobe to pullover tops and pull up pants or skirts. Forget the buttons!*
• *Wear clasp-less jewelry — slide-on bracelets and necklaces can be just as cute*
• *Invest in soft, wireless bandeau bras if the hard wires of traditional bras are painful to you and don't worry that they might not be as flattering. When you have a grimace on your face because you're in pain, you're probably even less attractive. (You won't have to remove them for X-Rays, either!)*
• *Use weekly pillboxes to organize your medicines*
• *Use lightweight plastic cups instead of heavy glassware. Your joints will thank you*
• *Alter your hairstyle so that you have an easier 'do with which to work. Don't you remember Julia Roberts in **Steel Magnolias**?*
• *Buy a wig if you're losing your hair or invest in a couple of cute hats. You'll save yourself the aggravation of trying to make those thin little wisps of yours behave*
• *Utilize a cane, walker, or wheelchair when necessary. Don't be embarrassed — hobbling around as if you're about to collapse is what calls attention to yourself. Breezing along with the help of a walking device does the opposite!*
• *Buy easy-open toiletries, groceries, etc.*
• *Invest in a letter opener for mail, etc.*
• *Replace your kitchen utensils with the easy-grip brands — they really make a difference*
• *Make life with pets as easy as you can — if picking them up is too strenuous, purchase an otto-man so they can hop up and down on your lap without your help*
• *Wear silky pajamas to bed, making it easier to turn over without disturbing your joints*
• *Swap out hard-to-turn faucets or door handles for easier turning levers*
• *Buy or request large print books from the store or library, if your vision is failing you*
• *Buy single-use packets of dishwashing soap and laundry detergent so that you don't have to measure out or pour anything*

- *Carry non-zip bags and purses, and empty them of all of the heavy items you shouldn't be lugging around*
- *Ditch the over the shoulder duffle bags and always opt for wheeled luggage*
- *Pay your bills online*

These are just a few of the ways you can begin to streamline your life with lupus. I'm sure you can expand on this list if you think about it. Go ahead – make life easier on yourself. You deserve it!

CHAPTER 7:
LET GO FOR GOOD

Obstacle #1:
my appearance

A month into my recovery from pancreatitis, my hair started falling out. At first, it was just a strand or two at a time, showing up on my pillow or in the shower after washing my hair. Over the course of a few weeks, those strands turned into clumps, and I couldn't even slip a shirt over my head without a fistful of hair coming loose. Even then, I wasn't too concerned. I had accepted that life with my chronic illness would (and needed to) change after my weeklong hospital stay. I had already reduced my hours at work, committed to napping on a daily basis and was taking better care of myself than I had in the past. I assumed the hair loss was just part of this transformative process that I was going to have to take in stride.

In fact, since my diagnosis several years earlier, I'd lost a considerable amount of hair on two other occasions. During those previous instances, the loss wasn't too substantial and stopped after about two months. After each episode, it wasn't readily apparent that I'd experienced any alopecia, as hair loss is clinically called. My husband and I could tell that my thick head of dark hair had diminished, but no one else would have suspected a thing.

Yet, this new hair loss episode was more drastic, leaving me with mere strands at the two-month mark. I started pinning my hair up in a bun to mask the obvious bald spots, but my hair became so thin that no amount of "comb over" could hide the loss. Two things finally forced me to admit the loss was abnormal and to seek professional medical attention.

First, the tiny, baby barrettes I was using were no longer holding my hair in place. It had grown too thin. I hadn't started with those mini clips, but had downsized from larger ones as my hair loss had progressed. I tried five different sizes before finally bottoming out at the newborn baby clips.

Second, Johnny, who checked me for bald spots every morning before work, suggested that if I thought it might help, I could consider getting a wig. He told me I looked beautiful no matter how much hair I had, but he knew I was nearing my breaking point. I was frustrated with the drastic change in my appearance and infuriated that the loss had continued. I was feeling violated and naked. When I glanced in the mirror, I didn't recognize the person looking back, and I was only 29 years old.

Because I'd consulted my dermatologist twice before, I knew that he would tell me to perform a painstaking, weeklong hair count, involving the following steps, as outlined in an instruction sheet from his office:

> 1) Collect 7 envelopes and label each with the date and day of the week for the seven days of hair collection.

> 2) Vacuum the floor of the bathroom and bedroom and brush off or change pillow case and head of bed at the beginning of the week. Clean combs and brushes and remove all hair.

> 3) Beginning at 12:01am of day one and continuing until midnight of each day, or for any other 24 hour period (e.g. bedtime to next bedtime), collect all hairs that fall from scalp and place in an envelope for that day. Remember to check combs, brushes, pillow, shower, sink, drain, collars, etc.

> 4) Mark the envelopes on the days of shampooing with an "s" or the word "shampoo."

> 5) At the end of the week, clean off a table with a bright light and contrasting background. Open each envelope individually, count the number of hairs, and write it on the outside of the envelope. Put the hairs back in the envelope and seal it.

> 6) Bring the envelopes to your next appointment for your doctor to evaluate.[1]

Also noted on the sheet was the following:

We recognize this is not exact but it is economical. It does give us a rough idea of the degree of hair loss. A normal daily hair loss count is up to 50-100 hairs, and up to 150-200 on shampoo days. Our bodies replace that many hairs each day.[2]

During my past bouts, I averaged a loss of 200 hairs on days I didn't shampoo my hair, and 350 hairs on the days I did. It was a significant increase from what is considered normal, but my doctor assured me that it wasn't cause for concern. However, when I performed this third hair count, I was losing between 500-600 hairs a day. I lost even more on the days I shampooed, although I had stopped washing my hair in the traditional sense. I just created a lather of suds in my hands and then patted it onto the few brave strands that remained.

The results of the count revealed what I had suspected: I was losing an inordinate amount of hair and losing it quickly. I'd waited almost three full months before seeking my dermatologist's opinion, so by the time I saw him, I had lost most of the hair on my head. The doctor and I went over the medication I was taking, hoping to eliminate any prescriptions with hair loss as a known side-effect. We also discussed several options for stimulating hair growth (cortisone or other drug treatments), none of which seemed ideal given the amount of medication I was taking already. He proceeded with a physical exam of my hair follicles looking through a super-powered, magnifying eye glass attached to his head. Lo and behold, what did he see but new hair growth on various parts of my head! He had to look through a crazy contraption to see it, but he firmly believed that my hair loss was nearing its end, particularly because there weren't any residual lesions or scabs, which indicate chronic, lupus-induced hair loss[3].

Because this new growth indicated that there was no further treatment needed, all I could do was sit back and wait for my hair to grow. But what was I to do with the dozens of stringy strands on my head? Once the stubble hairs grew longer, I was really going to look silly. As I contemplated my options, I realized that I was grasping at those long, wispy strands because they were my final attempt to hold onto the person I was before being diagnosed with lupus. I never expected my stubbornness and determination to manifest themselves in the way I viewed my physical appearance, but they were, and I needed to figure out a way to deal with them.

This was yet another turning point for me, a stepping stone along the path to wellness. It was an opportunity to put aside my past expectations, this time, of what I should look like. Just because I'd always had thick, long dark hair in the past didn't mean it was an essential part of who I was today. Instead of preserving an old identity that no longer existed, I needed to focus on creating a new version of myself, one that would reflect my new attitude toward life with a chronic illness. In fact, as I stared at my balding head, I realized I had no choice.

> ❝ *The greatest discovery of my generation is that human beings can alter their lives by altering their attitudes of mind.* [4]

Convinced that the time had come to finally let go, I grabbed the phone book, turned to the section on hair salons, and found the name of a place I passed a few times in the mall. My regular hair stylist was away on a month's vacation, but if I didn't act now, I might lose the courage to do so later. I placed a call to the random salon and made an appointment to have my hair chopped off by one of their "short hair experts", who, I was told, would "totally know what to do."

As I headed out the door for my appointment, I caught sight of my reflection in the hallway mirror. Somehow, I already looked different. Maybe it was the relief of finally doing something proactive about the consequences of having lupus. Maybe it was the swell of confidence that had come over me as I'd made the call. Whatever it was, I knew a major change was occurring. The change was coming about, not just because I was getting a new hairdo, but also because I was taking steps to cut out the hurt, anger, and resentment I'd carried around over the last three years with lupus. I was relinquishing the hold I had on my past life, and letting go felt great!

The details of my hair-cut with Ty, my stylist, were somewhat uneventful, although I can say that he was one of the more colorful, uninhibited, albeit compassionate, people I've met. With my sister by my side, I explained my situation to him: the disease, the hair loss, and the recent hair growth that was barely there. His nods of comprehension made it seem as if he worked with balding, stringy-haired clients every day. He was encouraging and respectful, just what I would expect from an old friend. There was no pity as he cut my hair; he was simply creating his own little masterpiece. The details he shared of his personal life kept my sister and me entertained as he cut. Before long, he spun me around so that I could see the results of his labors. As I stared back at the face in the mirror, I was shocked. No longer did I see a face full of anxiety, dread, or burden. Instead, I saw a woman with a renewed sense of dignity and confidence. I had a sassy, super short, pixy-like hairdo to accompany my transformation, but as I looked at my new image, I realized that it had been a long time since I'd felt so beautiful, inside *and* out.

Before I left, Ty asked if I wanted to "keep the tail," the strands that he'd pulled back into a makeshift pony tail and cut to begin my transformative hairdo. My sister and I took one look at the wet, ragged strands that now resembled a rat's tail, (and probably did when they were on my head) and just burst out laughing. "I won't need that," I said. I knew I wouldn't, not where I was headed.

I arrived home, and Johnny absolutely loved the new 'do. He thought I looked like a magazine model and immediately insisted that we have an impromptu photo shoot in the back yard. The loving, enthralled look he had on his face as he shot those pictures made me feel like I was the most beautiful woman in the whole world. He always told me I was, but I forever will cherish the captivated way in which he embraced me and my new haircut that day. After shooting a few pictures, he proudly sent them off via email to some family members, who all responded with the same complimentary remarks.

I continued to receive the same feedback over the next few days from friends and co-workers. While people decidedly were remarking on the haircut, they were also responding to the evident changes in my persona. Gone were my humiliation and self-consciousness, boldly replaced with courage and composure. I was no longer ashamed by what lupus had done to me. Instead, I could speak of the steps I was taking to manage its fallout. I was showing the world that lupus may have taken my hair, but it wouldn't rob me of my vitality.

Even though a short hairdo wasn't what I had ever wanted before, it turned out to be just the change I needed to jumpstart my stalled journey to permanent health and wellness. Considering that I had never before contemplated cutting my hair, I began wondering what other physical or emotional changes I too quickly had dismissed in the past. I thought of the outdated and unrealistic expectations I was placing on myself and my unnecessary feelings of guilt. As I revisited my life-long goals, I tried to make them more relevant and current to my life with lupus. I based them on what I could do, what I wanted to do, and what I needed to do to feel good, inside and out. I concentrated on making decisions that wouldn't just perpetuate my life, but that would improve it. I had been standing in the way of my final push toward wellness, but recognizing the error of my ways allowed me to finally let go for good.

The positive changes that took place during the months after I got my hair cut continue today. Still, I strive each day to maintain the healthy lifestyle to which I've become accustomed. While the decisions I face haven't diminished completely, they have become easier. Living well isn't something I have to work hard to achieve anymore. Today, it comes naturally.

In this chapter, we'll look at the steps that will help you let go for good. In order to do so, you'll need to re-evaluate the following three areas:

→ **The methods for getting what you want**
→ **The expectations you set for yourself**
→ **The sources of your guilt**

In doing so, you will make strides toward regaining a life worth living.

REEVALUATE...

REEVALUATE YOUR METHODS OF GETTING WHAT YOU WANT

Since the day of your diagnosis, you've wanted one thing only: a life free of lupus. You've prayed and begged for your chronic illness to go away, knowing that would be the easiest way to regain your familiar way of life. You may even have made a few bargains along the way, saying "If my disease would miraculously go away, I promise I'll never [blank] again." But frustration has set in because your wishes haven't been granted. In fact, it may seem like your pleas are being ignored. You wonder what part of "Heal Me" God doesn't understand.

Perhaps this is a better question to ask: what part of the puzzle don't *you* understand? Right now, you see a complete physical healing as the only assurance of regaining a life worth living. But what if a perfectly-functioning body isn't yours to have at the present time? More importantly, what if it doesn't solve the larger issue that looms over you – the long-term emotional effects of being diagnosed with a chronic illness? You're a different person than you were before lupus arrived; denying that is ignoring the essence of who you have become. The remedy for the hopelessness you feel due to your physical ailments may lie in an emotional contentment you haven't yet considered.

◊✑ EXAMPLE

After ten years of marriage, a friend of mine separated from her husband. During the months of separation, her husband refused to participate in marriage counseling and declined any sort of therapy to address his own personal issues of control and rage. Reuniting with her husband was my friend's primary objective, one that she thought was best for her family and her own happiness and security. But her hopes and prayers weren't being answered, and her husband continued to be uncooperative. Frustrated, she began to question whether her pleas for reconciliation were somehow misguided. What if the outcome she wanted and expected wasn't in fact the one that was planned for her? Thus, she began to put aside her presupposition of getting back together and, instead, started focusing on the inevitable. She took steps to plan for the financial and logistical changes she would need to make if, in fact, her marriage failed.

Her refocused efforts brought her immediate results. Instead of the feelings of hopelessness that she experienced trying to save a doomed marriage, she felt like she was finally making a difference. She felt prepared, confident and relieved. Despite the fact that it was a prospect for which she hadn't planned originally, she felt good about her progress rather than frustrated by her previous fruitless efforts.

I found the same to be true in my struggles with lupus. Every day for years, I prayed that God would heal my broken down body. I wasn't expecting a miracle, but I had come to believe that, if I were patient enough, I would get the physical healing I wanted. As the disease worsened, I grew more discouraged. *Why wasn't God listening to me?* Maybe I wasn't being clear enough. Or maybe it wasn't a healing I needed, but an understanding of what was realistically in my future. By changing my focus, my frustrations caused by having made such little physical progress went away, replaced with an appreciation for the emotional acceptance I instantly was capable of achieving.

❝ *Prayer is not asking for what you think you want, but asking to be changed in ways you can't imagine.*[5]

Instead of perpetuating the short-sighted, limited notions of how you can physically mend your broken body, start working toward that which can be realized immediately — a healthy acceptance of where you are in your life today. You'll no longer be chasing a hopeless, unreachable goal of living well without lupus. Your objective will become living well, *despite* lupus.

REEVALUATE YOUR EXPECTATIONS

One year, I made it a goal to become well enough to give up my perfunctory, daily nap. I had visions of regaining my previous level of functionality before lupus, thinking that the dismissal of my nap would be a good indication that I had accomplished this. I came up with three reasons why ditching my nap would be such a welcomed change. One - it would be nice to resume a full day of work. Two - I could book travel arrangements without considering when or where I would take a nap. Three - social engagements would no longer have to be moved earlier or later due to the timing of my nap.

However, these areas of accommodation didn't seem to bother anyone but me. My supervisor wasn't complaining about my shortened work schedule, my husband wasn't inconvenienced by the extra planning that was required when we traveled or made evening plans, and my friends and family had no problem working social get-togethers around my nap. In fact, everyone thought my daily nap had been a great addition to my life except me. They claimed I was healthier, more energetic and more engaged during the evening hours. Thus, I could no longer blame my reasons on the needs or convenience of others. And if I couldn't do that, did I really have a good excuse for ditching the nap? What harm was it doing me to rest for a couple of hours? Was I really missing out on anything? The answer, of course, was no. This was a self-imposed goal, one based upon my own expectations of what it meant to be "normal." But if no one else cared, should I? Should you?

While it's easier to blame the expectations you have for yourself on the whims

of a boss, your spouse, or the kids, take a moment to ask yourself whose standards you're really trying to meet. Are they someone else's, or are they actually
your own?

Next, ask yourself how permanent those expectations of yours are. Are they written in stone? I imagine they're not. You must be strong and courageous, taking
the proactive and necessary steps to rewrite the tablet yourself. The hurdles you
face in doing this don't lie in other people's perception of you and lupus; it's your
own scrutiny that needs to be re-examined.

Obstacle #2:
my plans for pregnancy

About the same time I cut off all of my hair, one of my primary lupus prescriptions started adversely affecting my eyes. I'd been on Plaquenil® for about a year and a half and, while I knew retinal changes were possible, it was such an uncommon effect that neither my doctors nor I were worried. However, my eye doctor discovered a change in my eyes after 18 months and recommended I stop taking the drug immediately. Because the changes to the eye caused by Plaquenil® are reversible, after less than six months of stopping the drug, my eyes returned to normal. However, I was left without one of my staple lupus drugs, and the prescriptions that I continued to take were not satisfactorily controlling my disease.

Dr. R suggested I try a new drug called CellCept®, an immunosuppressant being used to treat a handful of active cases of lupus, primarily those with kidney involvement. It was normally prescribed in combination with other drugs to prevent the rejection of kidney, liver or heart transplants. Because of this, I saw it as a riskier, more aggressive drug than the cocktail of steroids and anti-inflammatory drugs I'd been on, plus I worried about its side-effects. As with any immunosuppressant, there was an increased risk to bleeding and susceptibility to infection, but there was another side-effect, in particular, that I was having trouble getting past: the increased risk of cancer. Dr. R explained that this side-effect was highly unlikely and felt the benefits far outweighed the risks. He encouraged me to do some research on my own so that I could decide whether or not to start the drug.

In doing so, I discovered another major caveat of the drug: I couldn't become pregnant while on the medication. In fact, in the literature I found online, it was recommended that a woman of child-bearing potential starting CellCept® be required to use two forms of birth control to prevent pregnancy before and during the treatment with CellCept®, and for at least six weeks after treatment ends (although my doctor recommended waiting at least three months). The article online also suggested that the patient have a negative pregnancy test within one week of starting the medication. Clearly, CellCept® and pregnancy were not meant to mix.

While my doctor was eager to start the treatment, I wasn't so sure. I didn't know if I was ready to postpone pregnancy. I needed to forge ahead with this new attitude of letting go, but I put off making a decision for several appointments, hoping that I would experience some sort of enlightenment that would resolve the question I rolled over in my mind.

A few days prior to my next appointment with Dr. R, my mom called. She had met Brenda, a woman in my hometown who had lupus. Brenda was just a few years older than me, was diagnosed with lupus about the same time, and had started a new course of drug therapy about a year earlier. She'd come across this new "miracle" drug that was controlling her disease activity unlike the other medications she (and I) had exhausted. That drug was CellCept®. Brenda had experienced dramatic improvements thus far, and was hopeful that the drug would enable her to become healthy enough to fulfill her goal of having children in the future. As I pictured this woman I didn't even know, experiencing an inkling of hope in her fight against lupus, I knew this was the nudge I needed to start the medication.

I had been blaming my hesitation to start the drug on the increased risk of cancer. But my real reluctance was rooted in my refusal to put aside the desire I had to become pregnant. It wasn't the drug I was avoiding; it was the change to my lifestyle. I was choosing to ignore the solution that my doctor was presenting in order to protect my own agenda. When I looked at the situation objectively, I realized how little of a conundrum I actually faced. The case for CellCept® had been made: my doctor was recommending it, I'd heard a very convincing success story, and the drugs I was currently taking weren't keeping me healthy enough to get pregnant in the first place. What was I waiting for?

Though it's hard to admit it, life doesn't always go as planned. Thus, trying to figure out what you did to let lupus happen (or what you could do to make it magically disappear) is a waste of energy. The only control you have is how gracefully you accept the events that transpire. This comes by re-evaluating the expectations you have for yourself and by relinquishing the sense of entitlement you have over life in general. The following phrase can be a reminder of just how simple this notion really is:

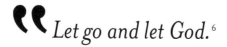 *Let go and let God.* [6]

You know some of life's questions are bigger than you are. Put "Why lupus?" and "Why me?" in that category and abandon your frantic search for answers that aren't readily available to you. Instead, learn to mold and shape your expectations around life's unplanned events in a way that will bring you peace, happiness, and perhaps the unexpected answers to your quest.

Earlier in the book, I spoke of a miscarriage I had years ago. I conceived in December of 2002 and had a due date of September 1st, 2003. I lost the baby after eight weeks and was devastated. How could this have happened? What had I done wrong? I desperately wanted a baby and, yet, it wasn't happening. Later that same year, though, the answer came to me. In the fall of that year, I suffered my bout of pancreatitis and landed in the hospital for a week, discharged on, you guessed it, September 1, 2003. The coincidence in dates was fitting, of course. This was clearly not the year I was to start caring for a baby. This was the year I needed to start taking care of myself.

Another mysterious yet telling coincidence came when my husband suggested that I start growing out my hair. He never had strong opinions about how I wore my hair in the past. Yet, for some reason, he made the recommendation. Less than six months later, the third bout of hair loss that I described earlier began, and I lost more than half of my hair. Because it was longer than normal to start with, I was able to maneuver the lengthy strands around my head to cover up the bald spots. The short bob I had before wouldn't have been sufficient at all. Perfect timing? I'd say so, but not by me.

Since life isn't always predictable or under our control, you must constantly revise and manage your expectations. You must accept your role as someone diagnosed with a chronic illness. In doing so, you enable yourself to live well and sell the rest of the world on your discovery.

REEVALUATE THE SOURCE OF YOUR GUILT

By the time I turned 31, I began to feel the pressure of not having yet had a child. By today's standards, I had plenty of time, but by my stopwatch, time was marching on too quickly. It had been more than two years since my only miscarriage and more than a year since I had started downshifting my life in order to get stronger and healthier. I was working part-time, napping daily, and watching my exertion and activity levels closely. I wasn't completely symptom free, but CellCept® had stabilized my condition quite a bit. Even so, feelings of frustration began to set in. If I was doing all this, and yet I still wasn't in good enough shape to start trying, when would I ever be ready? Was conceiving and carrying a child even a possibility for someone with my disease? My anger gave way to panic and desperation and, slowly, I started blaming myself for my present situation. I felt guilty for my failed attempts to get pregnant and for the years I'd "lost" because of lupus. I saw this waiting period as a direct result of something I was doing wrong. It was my fault that my plan of "kids by the age of 28" had fallen through.

Deep down, I knew my guilt was misplaced, but I couldn't shake it. I tried to convince myself that I was doing the right thing by taking time to get healthy, but I felt selfish and culpable. I couldn't dismiss my guilt-ridden feelings, no matter how hard I tried.

I started bringing up the subject with my husband, who was reluctant to discuss the matter in depth. He was in no hurry to rush the process. He was thrilled to have his healthy, able-bodied wife back, and had no intention of reversing the progress I had made. But, after several attempts to shirk my conversations on the subject, he had finally had enough.

One day, when I started in on the topic, whimpering and whining about how I wanted to change medications so I could start trying to get pregnant soon, he stopped what he was doing and looked me straight in the eye. Calmly, yet with a hint of authority in his voice, he said he thought it would be best if we waited to discuss the idea of getting pregnant until I was at least 33. *Thirty-three! That was two years from now!* While my immediate reaction was shock and dismay, within a minute or to of his declaration, I felt a sense of calm come over my body. I knew I needed more time to heal, but I hadn't been willing to give myself permission to take it. I had neither the patience nor discipline to tell myself it was okay to wait. Johnny had seen (and heard) the emotional angst I was causing myself. He knew the boundaries with which I was struggling, and he decided to intervene.

This involvement on his part, in and of itself, is a perfect example of the "growth" we both experienced over those first few years with lupus. In the beginning, he gave me free reign to determine my own boundaries, appointing me the keeper of my own health and wellness. He trusted me to make good decisions, and I felt confident in making them. But, over the years, he recognized how difficult it was for me to do so. I was too overwhelmed and stubborn to make some of the lifestyle changes myself. Deep down, I knew I was failing on my own, so he started offering me the gentle coercion I needed to make the right decisions, and I started listening. He ushered me into bed when it was time for my nap and insisted on take-out when he could see I was too spent to make dinner. He had always been supportive, caring and concerned, but now, he was fully engaged.

Because of his intimate knowledge and understanding of my unrelenting personality, he knew he needed to relieve me of my baby deadline. In fact, he concluded that he needed to issue one of his own. Together, we discussed the value of waiting, and he reminded me of the monumental strides I'd made up to that point. If I continued my efforts, my health would continue to improve over the next two years. We decided to enjoy the blessings of my restored health (and life without dependents), while continuing to be mindful of my health needs and accommodations. Putting leisure, relaxation and enjoyment at the forefront, we traveled the world, racking up ten new countries (following my travel tips from Chapter 6 each time.) We made plans to renovate our home and took the necessary steps to start transitioning me out of my part-time job completely. We both knew that "retiring" was the best way to keep me healthy, so we united our efforts and decided to make it happen within the year.

By putting the baby talk on hold for the foreseeable future, my guilt all but disappeared. It was replaced with a renewed sense of purpose and resolve. Working within the boundary of age, I was able to concentrate on getting as healthy as possible by the age of 33, without having to deliberate daily over the decision of whether or not I should start trying to have a baby.

The only anxious feelings that remained came from an unfounded assumption that my in-laws might be disappointed by my postponed or eventual inability to produce grandchildren. While they had always been extremely supportive and had never uttered a single word to substantiate my thoughts, I still felt like I was letting them down. Unknowingly, my mother-in-law squelched my unfounded conjecture one afternoon while we were on vacation.

She and I were chatting and the subject of children came up. She said that, when the time was right, things would fall into place for me. She went on to mention the success that some of her friends had experienced with adoption and noted that it might benefit me to start researching resources, just in case. Here, she was openly creating options for me, rather than judging me as I supposed she might have reason to do. There was no resentment or anger – she conveyed only compassion, support, and love. I knew then what I had always known: that she and my father-in-law loved me for who I was and accepted everything about me as if I was their own daughter.

To this day, the love and advice she gave me that day remind me of how mistaken I had been. In particular, it helped to stifle any further feelings of guilt I had pertaining to pregnancy. From that moment on, I knew that the only person fabricating any notion of blame was me.

You, too, must let go of the guilt that is self-inflicted. Just as you have before, you must focus your energy on the positive strides you've made in your life with lupus, not the areas you feel are lacking. My dad suggests "going to the good first," which forces you to make room for the things you're doing well while pushing out those thoughts of self-doubt. What went well in your life today? Name at least one thing that went right and then congratulate yourself for making it happen. Could you do even more tomorrow?

Even the culpability you feel at work can be addressed in a similar manner. Perhaps you're struggling with co-workers who can't seem to grasp your limitations. As long as you have taken the proper steps to inform your employer of your restrictions and are fulfilling your obligations as you've discussed, don't let anyone else shame you into feeling guilty about the quality of your performance. Judgmental behavior is typically the result of a misunderstanding – and as hard as you're working to live well, you don't have time to worry about someone else's misconception. Be confident in knowing that you're doing your part and let them come around when they're ready. You may feel compelled to educate them on your situation, but do so in order to achieve your own peace of mind, not in an effort to appease theirs. They may be struggling with issues of insecurity and self-doubt of their own, and you certainly don't need to take those upon yourself. If need be, consult your supervisor more frequently to reassure yourself that you're living up to the expectations that have been set for you. If you are, you should walk tall. If you're not, then at least you'll be apprised of what you need to start doing.

LETTING GO FOR GOOD -
putting it into practice

Now it's time for you to reflect on those things that are preventing you from letting go for good.

1) Focus on three primary obstacles that are currently standing in your way of living well. You may be able to think of a dozen right now, but start with the three that come to mind first. Think of these as the final road blocks on your path to wellness - you've come this far; don't let these stop you now.

2) As you identify each obstacle, jot down what is keeping these obstacles in your way. Remember, your reasoning is probably based on the pre-conceived notions you have for getting what you want, your personal expectations, and self-inflicted guilt.

3) Knowing that you need to overcome each obstacle in order to make the final push toward wellness, write down at least three bona fide reasons why you should remove them from your path. You may find that health and happiness are reoccurring themes in your reasoning, and if so, that's great! What better reasons do you need than to propagate your own well-being and longevity?

4) Now, make note of at least three action items you plan to take to remove each obstacle from your path. It never hurts to outline the stepping stones you have in front of you in order to see just how close you are to your goal of living well.

Now pat yourself on the back. You've just put the finishing touches on your blueprint for living well. Congratulations!

Of the three obstacles that littered my final pathway to wellness (the others being my appearance and plans for pregnancy), obstacle #3 proved to be the hardest. But by doing what I just tasked you to do: analyzing the reasons why I felt the way I did, evaluating what was standing in my way, and creating an action plan to overcome it, I enabled myself to let go of the obstacle. I had to go back and rework several steps mentioned in this book, but it was worth it.

Obstacle #3:
my job

In the spring of 2006, I decided to stop working completely. Three years earlier, I opted to reduce my work week to 32 hours, working one day from home to accommodate my ailing health. I was still in a management position, but slowly, it became obvious that my body could no longer tolerate the stress that accompanied it. A year later, I chose to resign from that taxing management position and work part-time from home as an associate in my department. It was an entry-level job, but it was just what I needed to regain an edge on my health.

Downshifting to part-time had improved my health, and I knew that full retirement was the key to maintaining my recently resurrected, active and enjoyable lifestyle. As it was, I'd started focusing on what was most critical in my life: stabilizing my health and enjoying my family again. I knew that quitting my job and having my days completely free would bring me even greater satisfaction.

Still, it was a difficult and heart-wrenching decision, filled with deliberation and uneasiness. From a financial standpoint, Johnny and I had some obstacles to overcome, but we were both determined not to let the burdens of insurance and other costly outlays come in the way of our happiness. Even though changes to our spending were inevitable, Johnny was doing everything he could to enable me to make my decision guilt-free. In fact, he had posted a list of goals on his computer about 18 months prior, one of which was, "Enable Sara to quit working by 'X' date." He'd changed the date a couple of times, primarily because I hadn't been ready yet. Johnny just patiently waited, fielding my bouts of indecision and encouraging me to think it through. I kept asking myself what was so hard about the decision. After all, it was just a job. Or was it?

I'd spent the last ten years putting my heart and soul into my career. I had been intent on doing my part to make the company run as smoothly as possible, putting other people's problems ahead of mine, and striving each day to make a difference. I thrived on the responsibility and the challenge that work brought me every day, and I wasn't convinced a sufficient replacement existed outside of a normal working environment. I felt important at work, but more significantly, I felt needed. In our society, there is a tendency to build up one's career identity so that the reason for being becomes intertwined with our reason for working. It's a natural entanglement, but a dangerous one when your health and well-being are dependent upon your ability to separate the two.

The dedication I felt for my work wasn't just something I could toss aside. I'd expected that giving up the managerial aspects of my first job would be a difficult adjustment to make, but I was surprisingly challenged in my new part-time position. My co-workers still made me feel like I was an integral part of the team, like I was really contributing. After a few months of feeling better without the added stress, I knew I'd made the right decision. I was still expected to produce and excel at my job, so I still felt accomplished. I just couldn't imagine how I could ever derive that same satisfaction from simply "being at home."

I appreciated that I was fortunate to contemplate the idea of not working at all. But I couldn't get past the fact that I would be 32 years old, with no kids, and no prospects for being gainfully employed ever again. What would I say to people when they asked what I did for a living? How would it make me feel when I responded or when they were left speechless after I told them the truth? I'd never felt inadequate about who I was before. But suddenly, I realized I was creating a situation in which that might happen. Why would I choose to do that to myself, especially after obtaining a good education to pursue my career? I needed and wanted to work hard. How could I just throw that all away? The anxiety of not knowing what would remain of me after I rid myself of this aspect of my life was frightening. Then I reminded myself of the lessons I'd learned earlier in my struggles: *I am not what I do, and my life isn't comprised of only one aspect.*

While it was daunting to think about how I would view myself without the attachment of a job, I knew that I was worth more than that. I was "me" way before I had all of that responsibility and expertise. I had a lot more to offer this world than just my ability to multi-task, organize, and produce. I was funny, smart and creative. If the things that would occupy my time in the future were nebulous and unconventional, so be it. It was up to me to prove to the world that I could still contribute, even without a day job. Maybe this would be the ultimate challenge, a test to see what I was really made of. I've told you about my confident, outgoing persona. Could I maintain those qualities, stripped of my armor? You bet I could. And I was ready to give it a try.

REASON #1 ESTABLISHED, TWO TO GO.

Having concluded that I could still be strong, courageous and successful without a career, another issue suddenly emerged. If I was so tough and resilient, why the heck did I have to give in to this stupid little disease in the first place? I know, I know. Back to square one. But this is the way things work along the path to wellness. You satisfy one aspect of your reluctance to adapt, and then up crops another one. It's a constant fight, but I guarantee you, one worth staying in the ring to finish.

Why did I always have to make the sacrifices when the disease never did? Lupus never capitulated, and it was always such a bummer to kowtow to it in the first place. Letting go of my career was a consequence of having lupus and I hated that. It was proof that, yet again, I wasn't strong enough. To admit that, at a relatively young age, you are physically incapable of doing what the majority of the population can do is a terrible consolation prize. I felt like I was being forced to quit because my body couldn't hack the rigors of normal, daily life. And quitting my job would be giving up and admitting defeat. Ultimately, it would mean a failure to succeed.

Failure was never acceptable to me. I was most comfortable pushing my limits in order to achieve what I wanted. That's the way I assumed you got ahead in life, the way you excelled. I don't doubt that's how I came to be Salutatorian of my graduating high school class, a scholarship recipient at the University of Notre Dame, or Facility Manager of a company at the age of 24. Those weren't goals that I'd planned to achieve early in life. Rather, they were opportunities I expected myself to seize once they came into my line of vision. If I hadn't, they would have become failures.

I remember a time in high school when I ran for president of the Pep Club and, unfortunately, lost. I was shocked and devastated. I had many other club offices to my name, but as co-captain of the varsity cheerleading squad, I had assumed I'd be elected. Even more shocking was the comment a friend made to me after the election. She said that I probably didn't even care about losing this race since I'd won everything else that year. *Are you kidding? Why would I welcome any kind of failure?* She saw no reason why I would be fazed about losing and, yet, at that moment, my prior successes were insignificant compared to the failure I'd just experienced. All I'd wanted was a perfect election record – and I had to settle for one that was flawed. I felt the same way about leaving my job, as if that change would somehow tarnish my entire career, making me feel like the last ten years were a failure. Was it so wrong to feel that way? No, but here was another opportunity to put my prior introspection to work. I needed to remember that seeking perfection might not be the best solution. *Compromise has its rewards, too.*

I reevaluated the decision that was before me. The compulsion I had to keep working (and to show lupus who was in charge) was more detrimental to my health than the decision to step down from my job. The sooner I made that change, the closer I would be to my goal of well-being. And wasn't quitting my job actually a preemptive move rather than a reactive one? Didn't it make sense to act before lupus could strike again? By revising my plans for a career, I wasn't failing— I was strategizing. Opportunities for healing and wellness awaited me; I just needed to get over myself and grab hold of them.

REASON #2 DOWN, STILL ONE TO GO.

One final stumbling block remained, and that was my plan for the future. You can imagine what people thought when I first told them I was quitting my job. The first and most logical question – where was I going to work now? When I declared that I was leaving the workforce and going to stay at home, the next question that followed, "And do what?" Well, that was a good question. *What was I going to do? How was I going to fill the days and weeks that followed?*

In the beginning, I told people that I was quitting so that I could devote the next year or two to becoming healthy, with the end goal of starting a family. People were surprisingly receptive to that answer, but I sensed that they wanted a more concrete explanation, and truthfully, so did I.

As I continued to refine my plan, I began adding that I would be helping Johnny's company with administrative work a few hours a week. He and I agreed that when I quit, he would start delegating some of the more clerical duties to me in order to pursue more sales opportunities. I was certainly up for helping out, and it would provide a little structure to my week, which I liked.

I also began mentioning that I would be taking care of my niece one day a week and, as my retirement date grew closer, I even started mentioning the prospect of writing this book, which was in its infancy at the time. It didn't take long before I realized just how many wonderful things I already had lined up for my future, most of which seemed a whole lot more significant than what I was currently doing. Spending quality time with my niece? Helping my husband build his business? Getting healthy enough to do everything and anything I wanted? Suddenly, it appeared that I didn't have time to work because I had much more important things to accomplish in my life. Releasing myself from the expectation to work would allow me to do something I had set out to do: *prioritize my life so that my health and happiness came first.*

This concept was unexpectedly reinforced on my last few days of work as people came by to bid me farewell. While there was a hint of sadness about not seeing each other on a daily basis, there was no pity or sympathy for my choice to quit. They shared my excitement about starting this new phase of my life and were thrilled to hear that I was taking the bold, necessary steps to continue putting my life back together. They knew how vital it was that I make this life-altering decision and showered me with encouragement and admiration to demonstrate their support. Thankfully, by that point, I wasn't seeking anyone else's approval, not even my own. I'd already given myself permission to rewrite life's plan and I was pleased with my decision.

I will never forget the heartfelt send-off I received on that final day of work. As I walked out of the company's door for the very last time, I knew one thing for sure: my future of living well would be my greatest success yet to come.

REASON #3 DOWN, ZERO TO GO. MISSION ACCOMPLISHED!

Today, I have no doubt that I made the right decision to retire. My life is fuller than ever before, and I've never once regretted the change I made to my life's plan. Did my health benefit from the change? You bet! Within the first year after I retired, I eliminated the maintenance dose of prednisone that I'd been taking, reduced my naptime by almost 50% and, by the end of that year, saw my disease activity fall to a practically non-existent level. Thus, over the course of the second year, I transitioned my drug regimen from CellCept® to Plaquenil® (because the latter was safe for pregnancy) and did so without any disease flare up. Keep in mind that, years before, Plaquenil® hadn't been enough to keep my disease activity quiet, so the fact that it was working on its own was a major victory. Because the transition was seamless, three months after I switched medications, my doctor gave me the green light to try and have a baby. Three months after that, I became pregnant. Nine months later, I gave birth to a beautiful, healthy baby girl named Deirdre. She's living proof that the path to wellness is one worth traversing. My life's plan, expected or not, never looked so good.

I have no doubt that you, too, will reap the benefits of overcoming the obstacles on your path to wellness. Each day you choose to live well, the emotional pain (and, ideally, the physical struggle) will lessen. You'll grieve for your old self a little bit less, and soon, you'll be living a new, improved existence you never knew you could have. By the end of your journey, you will have a new appreciation for yourself, despite lupus.

CHAPTER 8:
LIFE AFTER LUPUS

Almost six years to the day after I was diagnosed with lupus, I found myself on a beach on the shores of the Indian Ocean, along the southern coast of South Africa. It was late-afternoon, the sun was just beginning to retire for the evening, and I was engaged in a backbend competition with my husband. There we were, frolicking in the salty water and luscious, white sand, enjoying ourselves as if we hadn't a care in the world. And you know what? We didn't. At least I didn't. For, despite lupus, I was living exactly the way I wanted to: traveling the world, enjoying a sunny afternoon at the beach, running and jumping in and out of the water without hesitation. I never thought a moment like that would come to pass — on a faraway continent, bathed in sunshine, feeling good from head to toe. I was agile, healthy, and symptom free — and, at that moment, I felt like the luckiest woman in the world.

Lucky

I consider myself one of the lucky ones. I'm lucky because I was diagnosed with lupus within three and a half weeks of becoming sick. I'm lucky because I have a husband who never once treated me like an invalid, as if I was letting him down or not living up to his expectations as a wife. I'm lucky because I have a sister who made it her life's mission to make sure I didn't work too much or sleep too little. I'm lucky because my mom learned everything there was to know about lupus, especially during those times when I wasn't strong enough to learn about it myself. I'm lucky because my dad solicited more prayers for me from friends, colleagues and perfect strangers than I'll need over the course of my lifetime. I'm lucky because my extended family and friends made it a priority to ask how I was feeling on a regular basis, letting me know they cared every day. I'm lucky because I have a one-of-a-kind rheumatologist, whose office will see me at a moment's notice. I'm lucky because I have two pug dogs who would rather rest in bed with me than fetch a ball any day of the week. (They're looking up at me as if to ask, "What does the word "fetch" mean, anyway?") I'm lucky because, when I realized that the stress, anxiety and long hours at work were contributing to the deterioration of my health, my supervisors suggested we revamp my hefty workload and demanding schedule to accommodate my health needs. I'm lucky because I have established a wide network of friends and acquaintances who also have lupus, each of whom readily share inspirational stories, words of encouragement and unwavering companionship.

Do I consider myself lucky because I have lupus? No, that would be stretching it. But I know I wouldn't have walked a marathon, written this book, or gotten my life's priorities straight had I not been diagnosed with the disease. Today, I see myself as living proof that life can be just as good as it once was (if not better), despite a diagnosis of a chronic illness. I'm a walking billboard for the health and wellness you can experience, if you allow yourself the opportunity. That happiness doesn't come without effort, but it does come with a renewed sense of self-worth and understanding. It comes with a more confident, secure, resilient outlook on life in general, not to mention a life free of pain, resentment, and anger toward the illness you have. Not a bad trade-off, if you ask me.

I feel privileged to have known the adversity brought on by lupus and proud to have overcome it. I don't underestimate the change that I've undergone since being diagnosed — I'm a more complete person having battled the fight, a more compassionate, learned, capable individual because of it. I used to imagine that, given my competitive nature, my demanding personality and my proficiency at work, there wasn't anything in the world I couldn't handle. Having battled life with lupus and come out victorious, I am now certain that there is not.

Besides a life worth living and the opportunity to do anything and everything I set my mind to, I've gained a few other things along my path to living well, which I've included on the following pages:

An appreciation

I've always been a relatively happy person, but I had never experienced true gratitude until I was forced to choose health and happiness over everything else. Despite the fact that I had temporarily lost, among other things, my mobility, my
hair, and my career, I came to understand that my reason for being was rooted
not in those tangible aspects of life, but in my ability to find happiness in the
intangible – in laughter, creativity, camaraderie, compassion, forgiveness, and
understanding. Finding the value in these areas of life allowed me to explore the
wonderful ways in which I can continue to contribute, despite the loss of that
which I thought made me the person I was. I never realized how much I had left
until what I thought I owned was taken from me.

" *Tho' much is taken, much abides.* [1]

Today, I have an appreciation for the little things accomplished in life: kneel-
ing down to pick up my dog, pulling open a door on my own, or jogging after the
post-man to get a letter in the mail. Just as much as I value those obvious signs
of mobility, I cherish the fact that I was able to carry on in times when I couldn't
kneel, pull or jog. It reminds me of how far I've come and how much I have to be
thankful for today.

An attitude

When I embarked upon living well with lupus, my mission wasn't to realign my priorities, reassess my goals, or revise my life's plan. I just wanted to feel better, and I was committed to doing whatever was required in order to accomplish that goal. The reassessment I did along the way allowed me to reach the greatest sense of self-awareness I have ever experienced, a consciousness that reminds me of how unique, worthy and significant I truly am.

> **❝** *I think the greatest blessing [lupus] has brought into my life is a sense of what I am worth.* [2]

I've had the opportunity to show the world what I'm made of, which is not only measured by what I can accomplish, but more so by what I cannot. It's in my willingness to accept the latter that my true merit is revealed.

An acceptance

Because of the rather displeasing scars that lupus can leave behind - skin rashes, swollen lips, and hair loss, to name a few - I've spent a fair amount of time on the receiving end of snickers, sneers, and stares from people who simply don't understand my predicament. But just as often, I've been the recipient of accepting glances, acts of compassion, and words of kindness from people who go out of their way to reassure me that it's okay to look or feel the way I do. It's this warm and understanding reception I've received from friends, family and strangers alike that has led me to a new level of acceptance today.

I'm less judgmental than I was before I was thrown into the world of lupus, primarily because people have been less judgmental of me. Where I once thought that others were at fault for letting their life spin out of control (not staying fit or struggling to keep a job), I now understand that sometimes, life just spins uncontrollably on its own. You can do your best to stop it, but you may never be able to do so. Perhaps I was afraid this would happen to me – and so, out of fear, I scoffed at the imperfections of others and catalogued them as their own personal failure. But it wasn't until my *own* life spun out of control that I realized just how comforting it is to be showered, not with condemnation or disapproval, but with unconditional support and understanding. It was the benevolence others showed me that helped my recklessly spinning world begin to slow and allowed my body and mind to begin to heal.

❝ *Heal me if you want,*
but take away my fear.[3]

Shedding my selfish fears caused my unfounded biases to fall by the wayside. I realized people deserved the benefit of my doubt, rather than my misappropriated judgment. May I continue to treat people as kindly and compassionately as they have treated me, especially in those times of desperation.

A purpose

Michael J. Fox, successful actor and long-time sufferer of Parkinson's disease, once remarked that there is no proverbial "vacuum" when it comes to managing life with a chronic illness:

> 66 *There's no vacuum – if you lose something, it will be filled with something else. So the lack of spontaneity has been replaced by the chance to consider what I'm going to do. If it's tough to leap, then you've got to look before you leap. Before, I might have just leaped.*[4]

As anxious and bewildered as I was about what my future with lupus would hold, I now see that as I was navigating the treacherous road of living with lupus, I was forging a path for my future. For with the knowledge and experience I gained through my trials came the opportunity to share my expertise with others suffering as I did. As I've learned about medical procedures that I could once hardly pronounce, health concerns I thought were myths, and insurance issues that I saw as insignificant, I've become better equipped to help others find their way through the maze of life with a chronic illness.

Each area of enlightenment has made me more attuned to my needs and to those around me. Although I know such expertise would have been a valuable asset during my days as a manager, I now feel an even more important obligation to share what I've learned with others who are in the same critical situation in which I found myself not so long ago.

Enjoying the new you

Now it's time to get out there and enjoy your newly discovered health and happiness. You have a brighter outlook and a more balanced approach to life with lupus; start taking advantage of it!

Keep in mind, of course, the small choices you made along the way that culminated in the lifelong decision to live well with lupus. Because you're better equipped than you once were, your deliberation over such decisions won't be as angst-ridden as it once was. But don't underestimate the choices you still have in front of you. Despite all of the great progress you've made, realize that living well is a journey that involves making good, healthy choices every day of your life.

When I started compiling ideas for this book, gathering my thoughts and putting pen to paper, I struggled to find the right words to accurately describe my current relationship with lupus. It wasn't that I wasn't living well. To the contrary, I had never felt better. I was six years into my life with lupus - I had retired from my job, was taking good care of myself, and had been symptom free for months. My disease was definitely under control, responding well to my medication and to my relaxing, stress-free lifestyle. Therefore, based upon the progress I'd made, couldn't I claim that I had conquered the disease? Weren't all of the difficult decisions of health and wellness behind me? Because I struggled to clearly answer these questions, I was never satisfied addressing the subject of "Lupus and Me Now." Thus, I decided to leave the topic until the end of the writing process, hoping the answers to my questions would reveal themselves in time.

Surprisingly, I found the answers I was looking for one day while I was waiting for my car to be inspected at a local gas station. I'd brought along a book to pass the time while I waited, but after a few minutes of reading, my eyelids started to droop and my vision grew blurry. Glancing up at the clock through my half-opened eyes, I realized it was time for my daily nap. I guessed this was going to be my last stop before heading home, where, no doubt, my dogs would be awaiting our afternoon resting ritual.

Yet, as I sat in the gas station that day, knowing I needed to take the kind of nap I had taken every day for the past three years, I glanced at the list of errands I had planned to accomplish that afternoon, and I was torn. *Maybe I could just swing by the grocery store on the way home to pick up a few things for dinner and then fit in a quick nap. But if I'm going to be that close to the drugstore, maybe I should pick up the film I'd dropped off to be developed; I'll still have time for a 45-minute snooze. And if I'm already there, I might as well shop for the toiletries I knew we needed. I could still get 30 minutes in before our evening plans.*

And, that's when it hit me – among the gas pumps and the oil cans– that my current life with lupus wasn't all that different than it was before. The tough choices I had to make to continue living well with lupus weren't past tense; it wasn't a battle that I had simply waged and won. Yes, I'd made a lot of progress, but my desire to live well was an ongoing process that was very much a part of the present. In order to avoid that terrible transition from a normal, functioning adult to exhausted, cranky, eyes-glazed-over lupus patient, I needed to head directly for home. But that stubborn, determined self wanted desperately to finish all of those errands on my list, despite what common sense told me to do. At that very moment, I was trying to convince myself to do the right thing even after years of being on the path to wellness.

In the end, I made the mature decision to go home and take a nap. It was hard being responsible, but I knew my commitment to living well shouldn't be ignored for the sake of some silly toiletries. I could hardly keep my eyes open anyway – was it safe for me to be running around town? I don't think so!

Each day, I experience less self-imposed resistance when I head off for a nap. Somewhere along my journey, the benefits of mentally and physically recharging have become abundantly clear, such that I no longer resent the fact that I have to take time out of my day to revive myself. My nap is no longer a hindrance, but an opportunity to relax and renew my fatigued body. Where I used to anticipate a mental struggle every day around 4:00 pm, my nap is now one of my most natural and accepted routines.

So, too, will your choices to live well become natural and accepted routines. You have what it takes to make the right decisions - simply remind yourself each morning of the commitment you've made. Look in the mirror at the healthier, happier, transformed face staring back. That should be motivation enough to make the choices necessary to continue to live well each and every day.

The unexpected journey

A young woman decides she'd like to spend time traveling abroad in Italy. She researches all of the right places to visit and buys her plane ticket. She takes a language course in Italian to become proficient and signs up for a cooking class so that she can appreciate fine Italian cooking. She reads up on the great works of Italian art, culture, and history, becoming somewhat of an aficionado in all things Italian. She boards the plane and settles in for her much-anticipated trip abroad. She dozes off and wakes up as the plane is touching down. The pilot comes over the loudspeaker and says, "Ladies and gentlemen, it is my pleasure to welcome you to Holland." "Holland!", she exclaims. "Why are we in Holland?" She doesn't understand how this could have happened. Her plan was to land in Italy. She knows nothing about Holland: she doesn't understand the language, has no appreciation for the art or history, and doesn't like the food. The airline apologizes for the mistake, but regrettably can offer no further assistance; Holland is where they landed.

What is she to do? She can kick and scream, demanding that the situation be resolved. She could waste valuable vacation time and money trying to right the injustice. She could refuse to leave the airport until she is re-routed to her original destination, no matter how long it takes. Or, she could adjust to her surroundings, learn a few things about the country, and attempt to live well for the short time she has in this new, foreign land in which she's found herself.[5]

You have lupus? Welcome to Holland.

Life with a chronic illness isn't something you could have planned for, nor is it anything you would have expected. But now that you're here, you have a choice to make.

Despite lupus, will you choose well?

Appendix

EXAMPLE OF CHRONIC CONTROL CHART, CREATED IN EXCEL™:

	A	B	C	D	E	F	
35		16	17	18	19	20	
36	SYMPTOMS:						
37	Joint Pain						
38	Chest Pain						
39	Throat/Glands						
40	Joint Swelling						
41	Angiodema						
42	Breakout						
43	Digestive Problems						
44	Fatigue						
45	Menstrual Cycle						
46	Vomiting						
47	Headache						
48	Weight						
49	LIFESTYLE						
50	Travel						
51	Hrs Worked (length, when)						
52	Hrs Slept (length, when)						
53	Nap (length, when)						
54	Exercise						
55	MEDICINES						
56	Prednasone						
57	Zyrtec 10mg 1 x day						
58	Zantec 150mg 2 x day						
59	Bactrim						
60	Percocet (Endocet)						
61	Robitussan 2 x day						
62	Tylenol 2 pills 3 x day						
63	Cellcept 2000mg x 1 day						
64	DOCTOR'S VISITS						
65							

August September Sheet3

EXAMPLES OF PRE-SCRIPTED RELAXATION TECHNIQUES:

[These techniques are] often most useful when you tape the instructions beforehand. You can tape these instructions, reading them slowly and leaving a short pause after each one.

· Lie on your back, close your eyes.

· Feel your feet. Sense their weight. Consciously relax them and sink into the bed. Start with your toes and progress to your ankles.

· Feel your knees. Sense their weight. Consciously relax them and feel them sink into the bed.

· Feel you upper legs and thighs. Feel their weight. Consciously relax them and feel them sink into the bed.

· Feel your abdomen and chest. Sense your breathing. Consciously will them to relax. Deepen your breathing slightly and feel your abdomen and chest sink into the bed.

· Feel your buttocks. Sense their weight. Consciously relax them and feel them sink into the bed.

· Feel your hands. Sense their weight. Consciously relax them and feel them sink into the bed.

· Feel your upper arms. Sense their weight. Consciously relax them and feel them sink into the bed.

· Feel your shoulders. Sense their weight. Consciously relax them and feel them sink into the bed.

· Feel your neck. Sense its weight. Consciously relax it and feel it sink into the bed.

· Feel your head and skull. Sense its weight. Consciously relax it and feel it sink into the bed.

· Feel your mouth and jaw. Consciously relax them. Pay particular attention to your jaw muscles and unclench them if you need to. Feel your mouth and jaw relax and sink into the bed.

· Feel your eyes. Sense if there is tension in your eyes. Sense if you are forcibly closing your eyelids. Consciously relax your eyelids and feel the tension slide off the eyes.

· Feel your face and cheeks. Consciously relax them and feel the tension slide off into the bed.

· Mentally scan your body. If you find any place that is still tense, then consciously relax that place and let it sink into the bed.

Toe Tensing

This one may seem like a bit of a contradiction to the previous one, but by alternately tensing and relaxing your toes, you actually draw tension from the rest of the body. Try it!

1. Lie on your back, close your eyes.
2. Sense your toes.
3. Now pull all 10 toes back toward your face. Count to 10 slowly.
4. Now relax your toes.
5. Count to 10 slowly.
6. Now repeat the above cycle 10 times.

DEEP BREATHING

By concentrating on our breathing, deep breathing allows the rest of our body to relax itself. Deep breathing is a great way to relax the body and get everything into synchrony. Relaxation breathing is an important part of yoga and martial arts for this reason.

1. Lie on your back.
2. Slowly relax your body. You can use the progressive relaxation technique we described above.
3. Begin to inhale slowly through your nose if possible. Fill the lower part of your chest first, then the middle and top part of your chest and lungs. Be sure to do this slowly, over 8 to 10 seconds.
4. Hold your breath for a second or two.
5. Then quietly and easily relax and let the air out.
6. Wait a few seconds and repeat this cycle.
7. If you find yourself getting dizzy, then you are overdoing it. Slow down.
8. You can also imagine yourself in a peaceful situation such as on a warm, gentle ocean. Imagine that you rise on the gentle swells of the water as you inhale and sink down into the waves as you exhale.
9. You can continue this breathing technique for as long as you like until you fall asleep.

GUIDED IMAGERY

In this technique, the goal is to visualize yourself in a peaceful setting.

1. Lie on your back with your eyes closed.
2. Imagine yourself in a favorite, peaceful place. The place may be on a sunny beach with the ocean breezes caressing you, swinging in a hammock in the mountains or in your own backyard. Any place that you find peaceful and relaxing is OK.
3. Imagine you are there. See and feel your surroundings, hear the peaceful sounds, smell the flowers or the barbecue, fell the warmth of the sun and any other sensations that you find. Relax and enjoy it.
4. You can return to this place any night you need to. As you use this place more and more you will find it easier to fall asleep as this imagery becomes a sleep conditioner.
5. Some patients find it useful to visualize something boring. This may be a particularly boring teacher or lecturer, co-worker or friend.

QUIET EARS

1. Lie on your back with your eyes closed.
2. Place your hands behind your head. Make sure they are relaxed.
3. Place your thumbs in your ears so that you close the ear canal.
4. You will hear a high-pitched rushing sound. This is normal.
5. Listen to this sound for 10-15 minutes.
6. Then put your arms at your sides, actively relax them and go to sleep.

Techniques reprinted courtesy of University of Maryland Medical Center http://www. umm.edu/sleep/relax_tech.htm

Works Cited

INTRODUCTION

1. The names of my acquaintances in this book have been changed to protect their identities.

CHAPTER 1

1. Hodgen, Barbara.Beamer. "Special Delivery." **Guideposts** Mar. 2007: 68

2. Livingston, Gordon. **And Never Stop Dancing: Thirty More True Things You Need to Know Now.** New York: Marlowe & Company, 2006. 127

3. Author unknown

4. Felton, Sandra. **How Not to Be a Messie: The Ultimate Guide for the Neatness-Challenged.** New York: Galahad Books, 1999.

5. The New American Bible with Revised New Testament. Mission Hills, CA: Benziger Publishing Company, 1988. 286.

CHAPTER 2

1. Kroening, Steve. "Staying on Top." **Success Magazine** Mar. 2007: 84-87.

2. See, e.g., Justin Kaplan, ed., **Bartlett's Familiar Quotations** 735 (17th ed. 2002) (attributing the prayer to Niebuhr in 1943).

3. For a specific example of my spreadsheet, see the appendix.

4. Angioedema: Swelling that occurs in the tissue just below the surface of the skin, most often around the lips and eyes. **University of Maryland Medi**cal Center. 27 Mar. 2009 <http://www.umm.edu/altmed/articles/angioedema-000011.htm>.

5. Suggested title: **The Lupus Book** by Daniel J. Wallace, Oxford University Press, USA; 4th edition, December 2, 2008.

6. Gilbert, Elizabeth. **Eat, Pray, Love: One Woman's Search for Everything Across Italy, India and Indonesia.** New York: Penguin Group, 2006. 187

7. Metta: How You Can Help. Metta Institute. 27 Mar. 2009 <http://www.mettainstitute.org/mettameditation.html>. [Excerpts reprinted from the book The Issue at Hand by Gil Fronsdal, guiding teacher of Insight Meditation Center]

CHAPTER 3

1. Livingston, Gordon. **Too Soon Old, Too Late Smart: Thirty True Things You Need to Know Now.** New York: Marlowe & Company, 2004. 50

2. Friedberg, Fred. **Fibromyalgia & Chronic Fatigue Syndrome: Seven Proven Steps to Less Pain And More Energy.** Oakland, CA: New Harbinger Productions, 2006. 25.

3.Proof. Dir. John Madden. Perf. Gwyneth Paltrow and Hope Davis. 2005. DVD. Miramax Films.

4. See Friedberg, supra note 2 at 50.

5. Robbins, Alexandra. "Confessions of a (Recovering) Overachiever." **Forbes.com/Achievement** 18 June 2007: 2.

6. See Gilbert, supra note 6 (of Chapter 2) at 171.

7. Moriarty, Helen, Editor. "Thoughts to

Sell By." **Selling Power** Mar. 2007: 106. [quoting Anna Quindlen]

8. "thrive." **Kernerman English Learner's Dictionary.** K Dictionaries Ltd. 23 Mar. 2009. **WordNet 3.0,** Princeton University. 23 Mar. 2009. http://www.thefreedictionary.com/thrive>.

CHAPTER 5

1. Livingston, Gordon. **And Never Stop Dancing: Thirty More True Things You Need to Know Now.** New York: Marlowe & Company, 2006. 84

2. *See* id. at 58.

CHAPTER 6

1. Alcoholics Anonymous Comes of Age: A Brief History of A.A. New York: AA World Services, Inc., 1957. 243-44.

2. Dorsey, Thomas A. **Precious Lord, Take My Hand.**

3. Bogert, Mac. Leadership Skills for Non-Supervisors. 2008.

4. Lupus Foundation of America: What Causes Lupus. LFA, Inc. 31 Mar. 2009 <http://www.lupus.org/webmodules/webarticlesnet/templates/new_learn-nunderstanding.aspx?articleid=2233&zoneid=523 >.

5. Green, Heather. "It Takes a Web Village." **Business Week** 4 Sep. 2006: 66.

CHAPTER 7

1. Instructions on performing a hair count. Alexandria, VA: Associates in Dermatology, 2005

2. *See id.*

3. *Lupus Foundation of America: The Skin.* 31 Mar. 2009 <http://www.lupus.org/webmodules/webarticlesnet/templates/new_learnaffects.aspx?articleid=2324&zoneid=526>.

4. Grinnan, Edward. "Editor's Note." **Guideposts** Jan. 2007: 2. [quoting philosopher and psychologist William James, as Norman Vincent Peale, founder of Guideposts, used to do.]

5. LaMott, Anne. "The Up Side." **Guideposts** May 2007: 9. [taken from her book, Grace (Eventually): Thoughts on Faith.]

6. Author unknown

CHAPTER 8

1. *See* Livingston, *supra* note 2 (of Chapter 1) at 82 (quoting Tennyson's well known saying).

2. Schamaun, Lauren. "I'm Still Me, Only Better." **Arthritis Today** May/June 2006: 16.

3. DeGrandis, Robert. **The Real Presence of Jesus in the Holy Eucharist.** Praising God Catholic Association of Texas, 1998. 46

4. Bennetts, Leslie. "Character study: actor and icon, husband and father." **Town & Country** June 2006: 198.

5. Kingsley, Emily Perl. "Welcome to Holland" **National Down Syndrome Congress.** 1987. 4 Apr. 2009 <http://www.ndsccenter.org/resources/package1.php>. [as told by Father Matthew Hillyard, OSFS].

Bibliography

Alcoholics Anonymous World Services. *Alcoholics Anonymous Comes of Age: A Brief History of A.A.* New York: Alcoholics Anonymous World Services , 1957.

DeGrandis, Robert. *The Real Presence of Jesus in the Holy Eucharist*. Praising God Catholic Association of Texas, 1998.

Felton, Sandra. *How Not to Be a Messie: The Ultimate Guide for the Neatness-Challenged*. New York: Galahad Books, 1999.

Friedberg, Fred. *Fibromyalgia & Chronic Fatigue Syndrome: Seven Proven Steps to Less Pain And More Energy*. Oakland, CA: New Harbinger Productions, 2006.

Gilbert, Elizabeth. *Eat, Pray, Love: One Woman's Search for Everything Across Italy, India and Indonesia*. New York: Penguin Group, 2006.

Livingston, Gordon. *And Never Stop Dancing: Thirty More True Things You Need to Know Now*. New York: Marlowe & Company, 2006.

Livingston, Gordon. *Too Soon Old, Too Late Smart: Thirty True Things You Need to Know Now*. New York: Marlowe & Company, 2004.

Wallace, Daniel J. *The Lupus Book, 4th Edition*. New York: Oxford University Press, Inc., 2008.

Recommendations for Further Reading

Armstrong, Lance. *It's Not About the Bike: My Journey Back to Life.* New York: Berkley Trade (Penguin), 2001.

Lewis, Kathleen. *Celebrate Life: New Attitudes for Living with Chronic Illness.* Atlanta, GA: Arthritis Foundation, 1999.

Quindlen, Anna. *A Short Guide to a Happy Life.* New York: Random House, 2000.

Index